What Your Doctor Doesn't Know about Fibromyalgia

What You Need to Know That Could Save Your Life

Linda Meilink
with
Patrick Rhoades, MD

iUniverse, Inc.
Bloomington

iUniverse Star
an iUniverse, Inc. imprint

iUniverse books may be ordered through booksellers or by contacting:

iUniverse
1663 Liberty Drive
Bloomington, IN 47403
www.iuniverse.com
1-800-Authors (1-800-288-4677)

Because of the dynamic nature of the Internet, any Web addresses or links contained in this book may have changed since publication and may no longer be valid. The views expressed in this work are solely those of the author and do not necessarily reflect the views of the publisher, and the publisher hereby disclaims any responsibility for them.

ISBN: 978-1-936236-34-3 (sc)
ISBN: 978-1-936236-35-0 (ebook)

Library of Congress Control Number: 2010917407

Printed in the United States of America

iUniverse rev. date: 11/15/10

For Lowell, who gave me the courage and inspiration to write this book.
And for Kevin, who was brave enough to marry someone with fibromyalgia.

Without compassion, medicine is devoid of its reason
to be.

—Arthur Rosenfeld
The Truth about Chronic Pain

Contents

Foreword

You cannot necessarily tell if someone has FMS (a common term for fibromyalgia. You will find both terms used throughout this book.) just by looking at him or her. Many FMS sufferers appear completely normal to the outside observer. This makes it difficult for many people, even physicians, to comprehend and believe the profound symptoms that many with FMS suffer. Friends, siblings, parents, and even spouses may feel their loved ones are embellishing or exaggerating their symptoms. This can be very difficult for individuals, making them feel like they are suffering alone and are without support.

The importance of this book is to help people to recognize both the severity and ubiquity of the disease. It helps individuals understand that (1) they are not alone, (2) their disease is real, and (3) they are not crazy. We do not have a cure for FMS yet, although we have medications and treatments to alleviate some of the suffering. These are detailed in this book. People need validation of their symptoms, giving hope in that they are not dealing with some imaginary malady but a real entity. If it is real, then it can be fixed, improved, or at least dealt with.

My personal opinion, despite the fact that millions carry the diagnosis of FMS, is that it is still widely underdiagnosed. This perceptive and fact-filled book will help patients and loved ones achieve the understanding and recognition they need and, consequently, receive better treatment. People can have rich and wonderful lives while carrying the diagnosis of FMS. I believe this book, with its empathy and education, will make a real difference in the physical and emotional suffering of those with FMS.

For those of you with this disease, know that you are not alone and you are suffering a very real disease with debilitating symptoms for which there is hope of management and improvement.

Patrick Rhoades, MD

Introduction

This book is the story of my struggle with FMS. After reading dozens of self-help books on FMS and chronic pain, I thought, "Someone should write a book about what it's really like to have fibromyalgia." Most of us, especially the newly diagnosed, feel alone, angry, and out of touch. I found most of the self-help books I've read, although helpful in some ways, were filled with the same persistently perky and/or impersonal tone that can be so irritating when health professionals use it to communicate with us. The books rarely touch on the angst and anxiety that we feel. Most self-help books minimize the seriousness of the syndrome. In many of them, FMS appears to be little more than an annoyance, some aches and pains that, with some medicine and exercise, could be alleviated. These books did not seem to reflect the agony and despair that I was experiencing, nor what I could do about it.

That's why I decided to write my own book, filled with personal narrative, humor and heartbreak, suggestions, and solutions. Most of all, it is a warning to other patients that FMS is perhaps the most widely misunderstood and mistreated condition that doctors face every day. As I talked to more and more physicians, I found more and more discrepancies in their theories and therapies. I suffered from wrong diagnoses, damaging treatments, and medications that made me worse or crazy. At the time, my inclination was to trust my practitioners. Unfortunately, FMS wasn't widely recognized as a real disease until the late 1990s. If your doctor was trained before then, what he or she knows about the syndrome may be limited and even wrong. I also hoped that spouses and other caregivers might read this book to give them some insight into what our days and nights are really like.

This book is for the lady who sat next to me in the beauty shop and confided that she also had fibromyalgia. It is for the young woman at Starbucks who told me her mother could no longer get out of bed. It is for the man standing next to me at the bookstore in the disease section who wanted to know if men could get FMS too. This book is for my sister, Darlene, who has bravely suffered from FMS for three decades, yet still manages to get joy and satisfaction from her life. This book is for all of you who are afflicted with this baffling disorder, your friends and family, and all those who want to educate themselves about FMS.

Chapter One

How Fibromyalgia Can Threaten Your Life

Just a week or two after I moved to Modesto, California, a fifty-six-year-old woman who lived near my new home died alone in a single-wide mobile home. Her neighbors said she once had a successful career working for the county health department. She had a good life until she was diagnosed with FMS in 2001. Soon, she was living on a disability check. She spent what little money she had on expensive vitamin and mineral supplements guaranteed to stop the pain. Then there were the stronger drugs, prescriptions for antidepressants, painkillers, and opiates.

I never met her. I drove by her estate sale a week after she died and slowed down to take a peek, looking for a painting or a wall clock to spruce up my new home. At first, I didn't even get out of the car. From the curb, the items didn't look particularly appealing. Then I saw her bookcase, which had been pulled out of the house and propped against the porch wall. It was filled with books on FMS and complementary texts on meditation, vitamin supplements, Tai Chi, natural food cures, herbal remedies, and suggestions on coping with chronic pain.

I recognized most of them, such as *The Fibromyalgia Handbook*, *Taking Charge of Fibromyalgia*, and *A Complete Idiot's Guide to Fibromyalgia*. They were on my bookshelves. They were the same titles, the same topics, plus a few I hadn't read. I got out of the car and climbed the four worn wooden steps. A round, gray-haired women was busy lugging items out of the small mobile home.

"Do you have fibromyalgia?" I asked.

"No, but the woman who lived here did."

She seemed busy, so I paid her seventy-five cents for three books and left.

"Be sure and stop back later," she said. "We have more books we haven't brought out yet."

I got in the car and skimmed through the books before I drove away. They were heavily underlined and highlighted. The phrases jumped out at me:

Save Your Money

Despite countless studies, no vitamin formula has ever been proved to cure FMS, so don't waste your money on expensive vitamin therapies. However, all of us should make sure we are getting all the vitamins we need. A vitamin deficiency isn't something else we need to cope with.

"Try to keep a positive attitude."

"Take time for yourself."

"Explain to family and friends that you can't do the things you used to do."

"The right foods can restore and heal your body."

From the highlighted items, it seemed her disease had mirrored mine and so many others. She also seemed to have approached it in the same way:

First with determination and resolve to get better.

Then denial as any improvement turned out to be temporary.

Then intense flare-ups followed.

Next came hopelessness as her doctor's previously positive attitude changed when she failed to improve.

Probably the office visits became shorter and more routine as her physician ran out of ideas and lost interest. She probably tried a different doctor or two. Then she searched for other answers, including acupuncture, chiropractors, vitamin supplements, special diets, yoga, Chinese herbs, physical therapy, biofeedback, and water aerobics.

Some FMS patients may get a little better; some may get a little worse. For most FMS patients, the symptoms will fluctuate on a daily, weekly, or even hourly basis. A baseline pain of two to three on a scale of ten at noon may climb to an eight or nine by dinner. When the pain decreases, it's easy for us to believe we are getting well. We want to believe it. We have to believe it. When the pain flares, I like to think that maybe it's temporary, and I start looking for causes. Did I exercise too much? Have I been exercising too little? Could it be a food allergy brought on by a grilled cheese sandwich I had for lunch? Am I stressed? It's an amusing concept actually. Everyone who feels like his or her body has been crushed under a heavy truck is likely to feel a little stressed. I spent nights paging through the self-help books frantically, trying to find something I had yet to try.

I spent long hours on the Internet. I subscribed to magazines. I went to support groups where everyone took turns complaining. I wanted to hear something other than complaints. I still wanted answers. I worked out. I rested. I went on strange diets and sent for vitamins that cost three dollars a pill. I realized that some of the medications my doctor was prescribing were addictive. When I asked him about it, I could tell by the look on his face that addiction was the least of my problems.

The pain woke me up at night; it was the first thing I recognized in the morning. It took over my life. A good day was no longer contingent on my husband taking me to dinner or getting that raise I wanted. A good day was when the pain level was low. Period.

The disease, chronic pain, and medication all interfered with my cognitive processes. One day, I was driving home, and I suddenly realized I didn't know where I was and

Sad Fact

Two of Dr. Kevorkian's patients suffered from fibromyalgia.

I didn't know how to get home, even though I was on the same street I had been on fifty times. I confused left and right. I said "Richard" for "Robert" and "crooked" for "cooked."

At some point, I recognized I wasn't going to get well unless researchers came up with a miracle cure. I started to think about all the diseases for which we have no cure: Parkinson's, Alzheimer's, and muscular dystrophy. FMS and chronic fatigue syndrome are just two syndromes on a very long list.

I began to focus on coping. If I could just get a little better, I could keep my job. If I continued to work out, maybe on good days, I would still be able to hold my grandchildren. I tried various pain medicines, often taking two together, but nothing worked for very long. My body rapidly adapted to new drugs and rendered them ineffective.

In the middle of the night, I sometimes woke my husband and asked him to walk the floor with me. My thoughts sometimes drifted to suicide. Research shows that nearly every FMS patient considers suicide at one point or another. The suicide rate among FMS patients is high. Although there have been no definitive studies, Danish mortality statistics report that the rate of suicide is nine times greater among fibromyalgia patients. I didn't want to die, of course. I just wanted the pain to stop because it was unbearable. I reminded myself that tomorrow might be better. It often was.

So I could trace the last five years of this unknown woman's life by the books she had collected. It took me about thirty minutes of skimming before I added it all up: the books, the estate sale, and the sad face of the woman who spoke to me. I wondered if the owner of the house had committed suicide. My curiosity brought me back the next day. As I stood in front of the bookshelf, the door swung open. The same sad-faced woman appeared.

"The woman who lived here, did she go to a nursing home?"

"No, she died."

"How old was she?"

"Fifty-six."

It was my age, exactly.

"How did she die?"

I knew it was a rude question. I just felt like I had to know.

"We don't really know. Her heart stopped."

She busied herself momentarily with arranging some articles for sale. She paused for a long while. "We're still waiting for the toxicology tests. The doctors had her on all sorts of pills. She might have just gotten confused, you know."

I did know. I had prescriptions in my medicine cabinet for five kinds of pain relievers, two brands of sleeping pills, tranquilizers, muscle relaxants, and an antidepressant. Just six weeks ago, I had been bedridden with a pain level of eight or nine on a scale of one to ten. My husband was out of town. The best part of my day was when I took my sleeping meds at night and knocked myself out. And, several times

> **Notable Quote**
>
> "Doctors now know that pain interferes with recovery; that it hampers an organism's ability to heal; that it brings with it direct consequences, such as increased blood pressure, and resulting stroke, heart attack, seizure, and brain hemorrhage."
>
> *The Truth about Chronic Pain*

when I held my sleeping pills in my hand, I had wondered how many it would take to kill me.

So now, I wondered if this woman, who was both a stranger and a sister to me, had been confused and taken too many pills, if she had taken them deliberately, or even if her heart had stopped from a heart attack from the stress of too much pain for too long. I felt sure that FMS had killed her.

As I stood on the sloping porch next to a table with electric massagers, tiny aromatherapy bottles, exotic vitamin treatments, and meditation tapes, I felt a terrible sense of loss and a significant anger at the medical profession, especially general practitioners (GPs) who see FMS patients every day, but often fail to diagnose the syndrome or refer patients to appropriate experts who might help them. They also discourage alternative treatments like holistic medicine, withhold appropriate pain relievers, and, on top of everything else, berate the sufferers for not keeping a positive attitude, going to the gym, or maintaining an optimal weight, as if the patients were somehow responsible for their illness. Worse, many don't believe in FMS; others who do acknowledge the disease often assume the patients are exaggerating their pain levels.

The woman who died on a Saturday night and lay on her bathroom floor until a neighbor discovered her the next day was only one of thousands for whom FMS was not a mild discomfort but a fatal condition.

Standing on her front porch in the weak February sunshine, I thought, "People need to know about this, the real truth."

Too much of the written word on FMS makes it sound so manageable that those of us who are unable to cure ourselves or, at the very least, reverse the disease and adapt to it look like malingerers or hypochondriacs.

As yet, there is no cure for FMS, but many patients, especially those treated by competent, informed physicians, will get better. Some (as I was) will be diagnosed with underlying conditions that can be treated. Others will respond to alternative treatments; some will have spontaneous remission. In these cases, doctors may never know why they improved.

For those who don't find permanent relief, dozens of treatments can alleviate symptoms, but GPs or other specialists in traditional medicine often do not recognize them. Unfortunately, right now, a patient's best hope for relief lies in self-education or consultation with doctors who specialize in pain or the growing field of specialists in FMS, even if it means that we have to scour the town looking for an appropriate doctor or traveling to get there. I have done both.

I have experimented with alternative methods and tried all types of medications, from Motrin to methadone. I have put together my own personal recipe for improvement. After years of suffering, searching, and groping for answers, my condition is stable. I am not cured, but I am much better than I had thought possible, awakening on occasion without pain, riding a bicycle, white-water rafting, and playing ping-pong. But, to improve, I had to ignore the advice of many, if not most, of the doctors I consulted and find what worked for me.

There is a real basis for hope. Some doctors are enlightened and can help us to get on the right path. Extensive research is underway; some of it has led to an increased understanding of the syndrome and how to treat it. FMS patients can improve. It happened to me.

I found a few health problems I could fix. It took a long time to discover them because, as soon as the term "fibromyalgia" showed up on my medical chart, doctors quit looking for other explanations for my health problems.

This is not to say that all FMS patients have underlying health problems, but they may have undiagnosed conditions that, when treated, will help heal the body and control some of the pain. They may have high blood pressure, heart problems, depression, hormonal imbalances, and an inability to rest. Their doctors may not be aware of how these afflictions work together, and they may not be up-to-date on the latest research and treatments for FMS.

But there is reason for hope. Researchers across the world have targeted abnormalities in brain chemistry and nervous system dysfunctions that will eventually lead to an effective treatment. Breakthroughs are on the horizon.

I was still suffering and without hope when I decided to write this book, the day I brought home the dog-eared, yellow-highlighted books from the house of a deceased woman I had never met. I could sense her desperation as I turned the pages, as she highlighted various remedies, every one a highly popularized course of action for reversing the disease.

I wanted to tell the truth about the hopelessness that FMS patients feel when their doctor's explanations and lectures fail and about what happens when you have tried every therapy in print and still can't control the pain. I was angry that conventional doctors had not diagnosed me correctly and ignored some of the early signs of FMS. When I complained of insomnia, wakefulness in the middle of the night, headaches, daytime sleepiness, aches, and pains, I think my doctors attributed it to the fact that I was female, menopausal, thin, and working at a high stress job. I was given antidepressants and Valium. I spent years paying for the advice of doctors who knew less than I did about FMS. Even after I was diagnosed with FMS, I spent hundreds of dollars looking for answers in many books that generally prescribed light exercise and a healthy diet.

An enlightened pain doctor once told me that she was confident that doctors would soon find a way to treat FMS, if they could only keep the patients alive long enough. At the time, I didn't know she would be one doctor who was right. Too many patients have been sent to their deaths by an absolute inability to endure more pain, aided by well-meaning, but ill-informed, doctors who failed to help them by dismissing their symptoms, withholding pain medication, and failing to do a complete search for underlying causes.

FMS isn't listed on a death certificate as a cause of death, but it can be deadly. FMS patients die from drug overdoses, lethal combinations of drugs, heart attacks and strokes caused by unendurable pain, withdrawal from drugs, and other causes linked to FMS. Sure, it would be easier for me to write that we are all going to recover completely immediately. Too many times, the helpful books I read (and there are some that were not) didn't seem to address the panic, helplessness, despair, and severity of pain I was feeling.

"If we can just keep our patients alive long enough to find a treatment," my doctor said, sighing as she handed me a prescription for Percocet.

This is the story of staying alive.

If you think healthy, positive thoughts, you will begin to create a momentum toward health and vitality. It is true. You can literally choose to be healthy, happy and successful.

Joe M. Elrod, *Reversing Fibromyalgia*

Chapter Two

Your Doctor May Be Dangerous to Your Health

The first specialist who evaluated me told me my health problems were mental. I hated my job.

"You don't want to work," he said.

I had been sent to him after an emergency clinic doctor diagnosed me with muscle spasms in my neck, bursitis in my shoulders, tendonitis in my elbows, carpal tunnel in my wrists, and arthritis in my hands, and all these various conditions began on the same day. I woke up on a Saturday morning in June 1999, feeling like a ball of fire had exploded inside me. I drove myself to an emergency clinic, where the doctor explained all these various conditions to me and prescribed muscle relaxants, heat for my shoulder, ice for my hands, electric stimulation for my wrists, and physical therapy for my entire body.

The clinic doctor's laundry list of diagnoses made no sense to me. How could I have developed all these problems in one night? How is it possible to get carpal tunnel syndrome and arthritis in the same day? For months afterward, as I made the rounds in physical therapy, I asked every health practitioner I knew. They muttered about inflammation, nerves coming out of my neck under pressure, work stress, and computer overuse. I had suffered from muscle spasms for years,

What Causes Fibromyalgia?

So far, there is no clear answer. A few doctors and scientists believe it is the same as chronic fatigue syndrome or a closely related virus. Others suggest it is caused by trauma (such as a car accident), neurological or anti-immune disorders, childhood immunizations, and spinal cord injuries. This list is by no means conclusive.

blaming them on my long hours at the computer. As the managing editor of a newspaper, I routinely put in fifty- to sixty-hour weeks. At times, my keyboard seemed like an extension of my body.

And everywhere I went, I asked the same question, "Will I still be able to write?" Then the doctors would suggest carpal tunnel surgery, electrical stimulation for my wrists, ergonomics, and a new device where I could talk and the computer would convert my voice to words on a page. After every doctor's visit, I cried all the way home. I had wanted to be a writer since I first understood where books come from. I was about five years old when I realized that someone had written the books I so loved to read.

"Someday," I thought, "I want to write things other people would read."

After several abortive career attempts, including a stint trying to sell insurance, cocktail waitressing, and a master's degree in English literature, I found journalism. It was everything I wanted a job to be and more. The first three months on the job and occasionally ever after, I drove eagerly to work, elated that someone actually paid me to talk to people and write about it. I felt a little dishonest taking a paycheck. I probably would have paid to do it.

Just a few weeks after I started my first job as a reporter, I interviewed a woman who had been in a mental institution since she was eighteen. Now sixty-two years old, she was about to be released for the first time. As I interviewed her in a tiny one-bedroom apartment, she leaned over and whispered to me in a childlike voice, "This is a nice place. I hope I don't get kicked out of here."

I loved telling the story of her courage, pluck, and wonderful sense of humor, and it earned me my first award for best feature writing, first place, from the California Newspaper Publishers Association, making me the star of the newsroom, at least for a day or two.

A few months later, I found myself embroiled in a state senate race. My newspaper, the *Paradise Post*, and the *Santa Rosa Press Democrat* uncovered a nasty little scandal, a senator who voted regularly on agricultural issues that profited a rice-burning plant in which he and his wife had an investment. This revelation cost the incumbent his seat.

Within eighteen months, I was the assistant managing editor of our paper, a small paper with a circulation of approximately ten thousand. Two old-school journalists, Lowell Blankfort and Rowland Rebele, owned the paper. They wanted to have the best paper of its size in the state (and one of the top three in the country), and they did. As editor, I often told people my job was to win awards for the owners and make them look good. And I did.

Of course, there was much more than the awards. I worked with entry-level reporters and watched them go on to jobs at places such as *National Geographic*, the *San Francisco Chronicle*, and *The Sacramento Bee*.

My children were raised and gone, so I could focus intensely on my career. I wasn't badly paid for a journalist. I had recently bought a five-year-old, three-bedroom, two-bathroom house in a nice neighborhood. Every five years, the owners bought me a new car. I had a 401(k) plan. I planned to work there until I retired. It was the happiest time in my life until I began my constant battle with pain in early 1999, when I woke up with the widespread pain that led to a crazy smorgasbord of diagnoses. Even after that, as tests were being conducted, I tried to ignore the discomfort, continuing to put in ten- or twelve-hour days. Never particularly fond of fast food, I used drive-throughs to pick up dinner because it hurt too much to cook or even get out of my car. But hate my job? Most days, I couldn't wait to get to work.

I was a poor kid. At my first job, I worked in a factory on the assembly line, loading cans of tomatoes. I had waited tables, pumped gas, tried to sell insurance, and stuffed envelopes at temp jobs to get where I was. I hated those jobs. I finally had one I adored. I felt I had earned it. It was my reward for a lot of study and work.

But now this new doctor, who had examined me about four or five times, didn't know me, and maybe didn't even know how I made my living, insisted my real problem was that I didn't want to go to work anymore. Wrong doctor. Wrong diagnosis. But the words cut deep. He had just told me I was a malingerer. Either I had a psychosomatic illness or I was a liar.

◆   ◆   ◆

My boss and co-workers might not have completely agreed with the doctor that I was suffering from a psychosomatic illness, but they had come to believe that I was just a little bit crazy. I complained constantly about the cold, even though my co-workers insisted they were comfortable. No matter how warmly I dressed, the constant flow of cold air from the air-conditioner on the back of my neck was excruciatingly painful. My hands would get so stiff that I could hardly type.

I went to my boss repeatedly, begging to be allowed some control over the thermostat or even have the editorial department switched to another, warmer room. I think my boss considered my complaints about the thermostat and my desire to move my office as an attempt on my part to take control over the logistics of the building. He ignored me.

I also complained about the music. Although our company policy manual strictly forbade playing music during working hours, the production and printing departments flagrantly broke the rules. The noise was a painful buzzing in my ear and in my head, making it difficult for me to hear on the phone and giving me unbearable headaches, especially when we were on deadline. The production department would turn off the music when I complained, but it certainly didn't make me very popular. I sometimes doubted my sanity, especially when background music my co-workers could barely hear irritated me. Did background noise really give me a headache, or did I really hate my co-workers?

But the insomnia was worse than the frustrations of the workday. I would wake up at 2:00 AM every night and lie awake for two to three hours. Then I'd get up at five-thirty to make my 6:00 AM aerobics class. I had been doing this for years. My family doctor told me to take Benadryl as a sleep medication, which often left me hung over and sick in the morning.

I sometimes fell asleep while talking on the phone to friends, especially at night. I went to bed at 8:00 PM most nights, sometimes at 6:00 or 7:00. After lunch at work, I would lock myself into a tiny office and lie down for fifteen minutes, not quite asleep, but not quite awake either.

Other times in mid-afternoon, I suddenly became so sleepy that I felt ill, almost feverish, although my temperature, when I checked it, would

Major Symptoms

Pain that is profound, widespread, and chronic and may include tingling, numbness, and burning

Loss of bowel and bladder control

Sleep disturbances

Mental confusion

Memory problems

Headaches, including migraine

Exhaustion

Irritability

Restless leg syndrome

Source: National Fibromyalgia Association (NFA)

be normal, actually a bit subnormal. On the days when my workload was lighter, I'd leave work early and sleep the rest of the day. I would sometimes wake up the next morning feeling better. Other times, I'd have to sleep for two or three days before I recovered. I'd sleep, wake up craving sweets, eat, and then go back to sleep. I often spent most of the weekend sleeping.

I called these episodes "the grunge." I asked my family doctor about them. He thought I was depressed. Even though I didn't agree, I started taking the antidepressants he prescribed.

By the time the pain showed up, nothing the health professionals were telling me made sense. My symptoms were strange and erratic. How could bursitis be related to insomnia? How could I have carpal tunnel some days and feel fine on others? Why did my hands hurt so badly when they got cold? What about those strange, flu-like symptoms that came and went every month or so? How could the pain travel from my shoulder to my neck and to my hands in a matter of hours? And how did any of that affect my stomach, leaking bladder, irritability, and inability to concentrate?

The pain was never-ending, sometimes searing and hot and sometimes dull and aching. On long days at the computer, it took every ounce of will for me to force myself to stay there until the paper was ready to go to press.

And the self-doubt worsened every day. I didn't tell my doctor about my sensitivities to cold and noise. I never mentioned my leaking bladder or irritability. I was afraid these strange and inexplicable symptoms would just further convince him that my illness was all in my head.

Hoping to relieve the stress that the doctor insisted was the root of my illness, I went to several chiropractors, a masseuse, and physical therapists. Some provided temporary relief. They all had different theories about my illness. One chiropractor believed my illness had something to do with vibrations from outer space. My Japanese masseuse believed it was karma. All of them lectured about stress. I sometimes believed the stress caused the pain. But in my heart, I knew the biggest stressor was my illness, and I couldn't get control of it.

If I had known I had FMS, I could have found books, magazines, and Internet sites that would have explained that extreme sensitivity to cold, heat, noise, odors, and touch is part of the fibromyalgia syndrome, as is poor circulation, which leads to chronically cold hands and feet. I might have known that sleeping problems are also an inherent part of the bigger problem. Certainly, I would have read about the inability to concentrate, or "fibro fog." I would also have found lists of other symptoms that included leaking bladders, irritable bowel syndrome, and even outbreaks of cold sores.

Oddly enough, the doctor who thought I was a malingerer continued to

Questions for Your Doctor

How do you diagnose fibromyalgia?

What do you believe causes fibromyalgia?

How do you think it should be treated?

How do you feel about pain medicine?

How many other fibromyalgia patients have you treated?

How did they respond to treatment?

How do you feel about acupuncture and other alternative treatments?

Do you believe fibromyalgia is overdiagnosed or underdiagnosed?

send me for more tests. He ordered some x-rays and an MRI of my neck. He sent me to a neurosurgeon, who said he didn't really see anything unusual. But because most of the pain seemed to stem from my neck, I still had hope that doctors would find something that could be fixed.

His final experiment was to recommend that I take two weeks off work. When I came back, I had improved. He felt that was indisputable proof that I disliked my job.

"Maybe you just don't want to work," he said.

I guess it didn't occur to him that most people, sick or not, feel better after two weeks of rest.

It's not uncommon for FMS patients to be told their illness is all in their head. When my sister was diagnosed with it in the 1980s, she was sent to a psychiatrist. Unfortunately, some doctors still believe most, if not all, unexplained pain is a psychological problem.

Did my specialist believe in the legitimacy of FMS when I saw him in 1999? He certainly should have. In 1989, the American College of Rheumatology recognized FMS as one of the most common rheumatic complaints, accounting for 10 to 30 percent of all rheumatologic consultations. In 1992, the World Health Organization recognized it as a legitimate illness. As a physiatrist, a doctor who specializes in treating muscle and soft tissue disorders, he certainly must have been aware of it.

I do remember him on at least one occasion pressing my back and arms. He must have been looking for tender points. At that time, FMS was diagnosed by the presence of at least eleven tender points, hard knots that are somewhat painful when pressed, located on all four quadrants of the body. I am not sure how many doctors rely on that diagnosis today. I know that I have them; other doctors found them. Did he know where to look? Did he catch me on a good day when I had few muscle contractions? Or did he catch me on a bad day when I hurt everywhere and couldn't distinguish one spot from another?

Or was he so sure of his own diagnosis, a psychosomatic disorder related to a stressful job, that he really wasn't looking all that hard for a physical diagnosis? Could he have ordered the MRI and the nerve study just to prove to me that I didn't have a physical problem? Worse, was he just making referrals to other physicians so they would continue to refer patients to him?

He certainly didn't believe I had FMS. But how could he imply I didn't want to do my job when it was obvious to all who knew me that my career meant so much to me? Maybe he thought I was crazy. As time went on, I began to think that maybe I was.

Sadly, many good doctors are out there. I would not tolerate that kind of treatment from a physician today. I hope that those of you reading this who feel your doctor is condescending or uncaring and unkind will find another doctor. GPs and family physicians may have a huge caseload of fibromyalgia patients, but few have any real understanding of it. Be prepared to shop around to find a compatible physician. Do not stay with your longtime family doctor out of loyalty or because you feel comfortable with him. Old slippers may be comfortable, but they sometimes smell bad, too.

GPs often have little training in pain management. In *The Truth About Chronic Pain* by Arthur Rosenfeld, Dr. Grace Ford of the Cohn Pain Management Center in Bethpage, New York, is quoted:

> [Chronic pain patients] have been treated badly because their doctors don't know what to do. I can't speak for all physicians, but a lot of physicians feel impotent when they don't know what to do to help and then they blame the patient. They think, "I'm a healer and I'm supposed to heal. If I can't heal you,

then something must be wrong with you—not with me." That's what we're taught in medical school, and if you have that mentality, then pain management is not the specialty for you.

Those with chronic pain need a physician who treats chronic pain. These doctors saved my life. When I was first diagnosed, I thought any GP could treat FMS. I also didn't recognize that not everyone expects the same qualities in a doctor. Some want a doctor who will listen. Some want to be treated by a doctor who exudes confidence, even though, in reality, he or she is concealing the belief that there is no hope for improvement. I used to find a good bedside manner to be the most important quality a doctor could offer me. I later began to realize I was wrong. I really wanted a doctor who would tell me the truth, even when it was, "I don't know."

Finding the right doctor may take a bit of shopping. I've visited several doctors once and never went back, but I know others who continue to go to the same doctor for decades because he or she is the family doctor who delivered their kids, treated their husband for basal cell skin cancer, and treated their daughter for pneumonia. He or she is like one of the family. He or she may not be effective at treating FMS, but patients will often argue, "He knows me." Doctors see thousands of patients over the course of their career. They may not remember a particular patient as well as the patient assumes. As a teacher, I have had former students approach me, and I didn't remember their names. And none of this personal experience with a patient makes a GP a specialist in fibromyalgia or pain management. This doesn't mean a perfectly good family doctor must be cast aside. But a specialist in FMS should be added to the medical team.

There are several ways to find a good FMS doctor, starting with the local telephone book. Many pain doctors will specifically list fibromyalgia as one of the conditions they treat. They may not know everything about it, but at least they recognize that it exists! Members of support groups for fibromyalgia or chronic pain may have several suggestions. But not all pain patients will appreciate the same types of treatment. A miracle worker for one patient may be a nightmare for another. Local pharmacists often make great recommendations. They know who is up-to-date on the latest medications and which doctors respond quickly to requests for refills.

One of the difficulties of our modern medical system is that many of us are in HMOs or PPOs in which the GP acts as a gatekeeper. Only they can give a referral to a pain specialist. I can't imagine why any doctor would turn down a request from a patient in pain who wants to see a specialist, but some do. I like to have a GP who will send me to a physical therapist, pain specialist, or any other doctor I think might be helpful.

But some patients eventually become caught between two or more doctors with opposing views. One doctor prescribes cholesterol-reducing medicine; another doctor is more concerned with the side effects of this medicine, for example, chronic low-grade pain. One urges his patients to keep working; the other fears the additional stress is causing an increase in blood pressure; a third doctor prescribes another medication.

My advice is that an FMS patient must pick one doctor whom they trust, but weigh all the suggestions that various caregivers offer. Remember, there is still no one treatment, so there is no reason not to try new ideas. But patients with more than one doctor must make sure that each knows what the other is doing so they do not prescribe a medication that conflicts with another.

Another serious consequence that can result from treatment by one doctor or ten is that medications become layered. This may result in the patient taking more medications than needed. For example, an antidepressant may cause serious headaches. Instead of switching to another antidepressant, the doctor adds another pill to battle the headache pain. This pill may cause drowsiness, so the doctor prescribes a prescription form of No-Doze, like Provigil or large doses of caffeine. These make the headaches worse. Soon, the pills are the problem. Need I say more?

At our clinic, when we see patients with fibromyalgia, antidepressants aren't our first drug of choice. We screen for depression before we start writing prescriptions.

Dr. Patrick Rhoades, director,
Central Valley Pain Clinic

Chapter Three

Why Prozac May Be Worse than Percocet

My family doctor believed in my pain, but he also thought I was depressed and antidepressants were the answer. In the past decade, I have had a love/hate affair with various antidepressants of varying chemistries. Some have terrible side effects for me; others have probably saved my life. I started taking them when I went to my family doctor for a routine Pap smear. I told him about what the specialist had told me, that is, hating my job. At most I had arthritis, which was dismissed as unimportant.

But I was frightened because my mother had rheumatoid arthritis. For twenty years before her death, she had walked with a cane or a walker, each step a painful victory. Her hips jutted out angrily, like whalebones. I used to rub her gently sometimes, wishing my hands could work away the crippling bone spurs.

So when the doctor casually said arthritis, I suspected the worse. Panicked, I went right from his office to the bookstore to buy some books to educate myself. From the books I chose, it appeared more likely that I had rheumatoid arthritis than osteoarthritis.[1] I believed it was rheumatoid arthritis because I felt ill all over, the pain wasn't limited to my fingers or knees or any other location, and I was weak and fatigued. So when I told my family doctor about the pain and my arthritis symptoms, I burst into tears.

---

1   This is good reason not to diagnose yourself. It's true that you should have the final word on how medications and treatments are affecting you, but, in the end, we do all need doctors we can trust.

He examined me, took my hands in his, and looked them over. "This isn't rheumatoid arthritis. See how your knuckles are just slightly misshapen? But they aren't swollen or red. Listen to me, Linda," he said as I wept. "You don't have rheumatoid arthritis. We'll run tests to make sure, to make you feel better. But I can tell you right now I'm sure that this is osteoarthritis."

Why hadn't my specialist explained all this to me? Concerned about my despair and pain, my family doctor suggested antidepressants. I had been on Paxil once before, and I had hated it. I gained weight, felt like a zombie, and couldn't have an orgasm.

Read All about It!

A quarterly publication, *Fibromyalgia Network*, keeps up with recent research and summarizes medical journal articles so they are easy to understand.

He told me that there were new ones and we'd try something else.

I can't remember the first one of maybe a half-dozen or so we tried, but they made me feel worse. The pills gave me severe headaches and made me want to sleep all day long. I would have no problems getting to sleep at night, but I would wake up at 1:00 or 2:00 AM and stay awake until 4:00 or 5:00 AM. My middle-of-the-night interludes were fraught with worry. Did I recheck the headline on page A-7? Or I'd have full-blown anxiety attacks. What if I never fell asleep again? What would I do if I lost my job? What if I had to go to a nursing home? Would anyone come to visit me?

Why antidepressants instead of pain medicine? I don't know what the statistics are or if any studies have been done to confirm this, but antidepressants seem to be a GP's first line of defense in dealing with pain he or she does not understand. Strong pain meds have to be carefully regulated while antidepressants are not. Antidepressants are less likely to be abused. If the pain is related to stress or depression, prescribing Prozac or a similar drug may be one way to find out. The relationship between pain and depression is still unclear. Even though antidepressants may not cure a headache or even a sore toe, they might make the patient less stressed and more able to tolerate the discomfort.

I was also taking Benadryl and Valium. Sometimes, in desperation, I'd take cough medicine or anything else I happened to find in my medicine cabinet that claimed to be sedating.

But the sleep induced by the antidepressants and other drugs was heavy and drunken. If I didn't have to work, I slept all day. I spent many workdays in a daze. For several weeks, I kept calling the doctor, and he kept changing my antidepressant prescriptions. Finally, we settled on Effexor, a drug that came in smaller doses so I could gradually ramp up to a full dose. I dutifully swallowed my pills. After a few weeks, I quit feeling so drugged and sluggish. I can't say I was any happier. The pain continued to increase.

Then something unexpected happened. I was offered a job in Sarasota, Florida, at a *New York Times* paper where two of my former employees worked. The editors there liked the employees I had trained so well that they asked me to come there as an assistant bureau chief.

One of these employees, Kevin Valine, had kept in touch with me since he had left the *Post* three years before. We spoke on the phone several days a week. Then we began to visit each other, and our boss/employee relationship had become a romance. We had taken a weeklong vacation to Key West the year before, a visit that left us with wonderful memories and a lingering question mark over how our relationship would be redefined. We had been lovers, but were we soul

---

Common Antidepressants Prescribed for Fibromyalgia

The EPA has approved Amitripyline, Nortriptyline, Effexor, Serzone, Cymbalta, Wellbutrin, Pamelor, Paxil, Prozac, Zoloft, Cymbalta, and a new pill, Savella, for treatment of fibromyalgia. But they are not a cure. At best, they will reduce pain by approximately 30 percent in some patients. Most antidepressants can cause weight gain. The benefits of antidepressants will probably offset the few pounds you may have to work at whittling off. Just don't blame yourself if you do start gaining weight.

---

mates? When I discussed my job offer with him, he told me he had thought it over and definitely wanted me to come to Florida.

So it wasn't a hard decision. I was desperate. I was getting sicker every day, less able to fulfill my job responsibilities, less popular with colleagues and co-workers, and more frustrated with my inability to accomplish the things I used to do. I hoped that working as assistant bureau chief would be less stressful than being the managing editor of a whole newspaper. I even hoped that maybe the doctor was partially right. Even though I still loved journalism, maybe I was worn out with the paper after twelve years. My boss had once told me that the average editor peaks after seven years. Perhaps my peak at that paper had come and gone. A change of climate and a change of environment could be just what I needed.

I had planned to work at the *Paradise Post* all my life, but my illness had brought me to the crisis point. I knew I wouldn't be able to do my job much longer. I had just returned to work after being off for weeks. My frequent absences annoyed my boss. Once when I had called in sick for over a week, he called me to tell me it was time to come back to work. That pretty much sealed the deal.

The day I told my daughter I was leaving to take a job in Florida, she told me she was pregnant with her first child. I had always promised to be there when she had children. We had planned that I would take care of the kids while she and her husband went on their second and third and thirtieth honeymoons. We would go to the kids' soccer games together. Now I was not going to be there.

As much as I wanted to change my mind and stay, I was more frightened of what would happen if I didn't leave. I was afraid of permanent disability, but I was more afraid I wouldn't qualify for it because even my specialist wouldn't support me if I applied for it. I would lose my house, my car, and my independence.

And that's just me. In any case, I never fail. I quit before I get fired. I leave before I'm kicked out. I fold my cards before I draw. At least I got one more chance, one more stab at an uncertain future before I bottomed out. I knew I had only a tentative grasp on my job and no other papers in the county would hire me if I were disabled. So I decided I couldn't stay in California. I was afraid that, instead of my being a help to my daughter, she would end up taking care of me. My move put more distance between us than miles could ever measure and, in the end, couldn't fix the problem. I would end up without a job and disabled anyway.

I remember driving to my farewell party so sick and dizzy that I wasn't sure I could wave good-bye. I knew I couldn't drive cross-country, so I shipped my furniture and car and caught a plane. Then I slept the whole weekend. I went to my first day at my new job exhausted. I had trouble following the simplest instructions while learning to use the computer system. Was it my illness or the antidepressants that made simple instructions confusing? Very likely, it was a bit of both.

Antidepressants can cause problems with word recall and concentration. For those who take antidepressants, be sure to read the prescribing information that comes with the bottle. Two of the mentioned side effects, confusion and memory impairment, can be quite devastating, especially if they are unexpected.

At that time, I know I began to suffer from "fibro fog," a condition that causes fibromyalgia patients to lose their train of thought, substitute one word for another in their speech, forget simple details like what they ate for lunch or what they were doing, or get lost on a familiar route.

I sometimes left the office to run an errand or get lunch and would end up completely lost and disoriented. This was unlike me. I generally have a good sense of direction, but, all of a sudden, I could not recognize familiar landmarks or put them in perspective. I had a map in my car, but, when I pulled it out, I had a hard time reading it. I would make a turn or two and find myself lost again. I sometimes asked for directions, but, once again, they didn't get me beyond the next corner. I blamed it on the pedestrians who had been kind enough to give me directions. They had obviously misdirected me.

Even though those of us with fibromyalgia call it fibro fog, FMS patients aren't the only ones who suffer from it. It's a side effect from living with chronic pain and a side effect of sleep apnea. The brain, as a pain specialist would later explain to me, can only take so much. Then it short-circuits. That is exactly what it feels like, like the mind blowing a fuse. There's just a big emptiness, a silence and a darkness where the words, thoughts, and feelings used to be.

My inability to concentrate, coupled with a dull, flat feeling, led me to make a huge mistake. I assumed that because my antidepressants were causing my stupor, I could discontinue them whenever I wanted to improve my concentration and, in general, feel better. No doctor had ever told me otherwise. At that time, many doctors did not know or understand serotonin rebound syndrome, a serious condition that can occur when people abruptly discontinue antidepressants. If you take antidepressants or you are considering them, I urge you to read the warnings and visit Web sites where former antidepressant patients describe their withdrawal symptoms. You will probably not crave the antidepressants when you withdraw, but the physical side effects can be life-threatening.

When I quit Effexor cold turkey, I crashed. Oddly enough, although my pain wasn't relieved when I started taking antidepressants, it welled up when I quit. Within two weeks, I rarely slept at all. I came home so stiff from sitting all day that I could hardly get out of the car. I had terrible headaches on the job and times when I couldn't remember what I was doing. Once I sent in a crime story without using the word "allegedly." It was the kind of mistake I wasn't used to making. I'm sure I probably made other mistakes that I'm not aware of, and I never had a good relationship with my boss anyway. And things continued to get worse.

Then I began to get these creepy feelings of electric shock on my scalp, usually accompanied by headaches. I thought I had a brain tumor or was losing my mind completely. I later discovered "brain shivers," as they are now called, are a side effect of antidepressant withdrawal, but I had certainly never heard of them and neither had my new doctor in Florida. I was reluctant to mention them to him. I was afraid he would think I was insane. I was also afraid I had a brain tumor. After weeks of working up enough nerve to discuss the shocks with my doctor, he brushed me off. My symptoms, whatever they were,

Flares

A flare-up is not the time to try a new exercise regimen. If you can, spend the day in bed, eat chocolates, and watch movies. Other ideas include:

Ice and heat packs

Acupuncture

Massage

Increased medication (with doctor's approval)

Listen to music

Meditate or pray

Soak in a hot bath

Remind yourself that this is temporary

Call a friend

Desperate Measures

If your pain is unbearable, do not suffer until you begin contemplating suicide. Call your doctor, or, if it is after hours, go to an emergency clinic. Under a doctor's supervision, you can be given intravenous medication that can provide enormous relief. If you have sleeping pills and clear this with your doctor, you can take a sleeping pill and sleep through the pain for a few hours.

had nothing to do with the withdrawal. Most likely, he said it was some kind of migraine.

Today, of course, doctors routinely warn patients not to discontinue their antidepressants abruptly, but they rarely tell you why. You have to be weaned off them, often over several months, to avoid the shock sensations and a host of other painful ailments, including headaches, nausea, dizziness, vertigo, insomnia, arrhythmia, and aggressive and impulsive behavior. I was naturally aggressive and impulsive, but, in the coming months, my aggression and impulsive conduct would surprise even me.

I will probably never know what my job performance was like in Florida, but my immediate boss, the bureau chief, and I had difficulties because we disagreed on some of the major premises of journalism. Nearly all papers have their own unwritten code about what has to be documented before the stories go to print or how aggressive a reporter should be.

Even though I felt I was on the same page with the *Sarasota Herald-Tribune* overall and I really admired the paper, I felt my boss was too careless in ensuring that all details were factual and presented in an unbiased way. I felt she modified stories to add spice where it was lacking. It was like being in a car with a careless driver. I was afraid we were about to hit a tree, and I didn't want my career to be pronounced dead at the scene. I finally appealed to the executive managing editor, who showed no sympathy for my dissatisfaction with the way our bureau was run. It was clear I would have to back down if I wanted to keep my job, but, instead, I did the outrageous, even for me. Shocked, outraged, hysterical, and in roaring pain, I walked out on my job.

I hadn't unpacked all my boxes yet, and I was already without a job. I told myself that it was okay. I had a sterling reputation, many great references, and plenty of awards. I didn't know that it would be years before I would write my next headline.

◆　　◆　　◆

When the word got out that I was looking, I got an immediate job offer back in California. I wasn't particularly worried about finding a job, but I did worry about finding a job I could handle along with the pain, insomnia, and electric shocks in my brain. Looking back, I sometimes wonder if I had committed career suicide at the *Sarasota Herald-Tribune* because I knew the fast-paced urgency and long hours in the newsroom were killing me. I decided to take some time off.

Since I had arrived in Florida, I had been living with Kevin. When I moved in, we were already romantically involved. After I arrived, I didn't look for an apartment, and he didn't ask me to leave.

If I had hoped that leaving my job would cure me, as my doctor in California had suggested, I couldn't have been more wrong. My pain swelled in the hot, muggy Florida summer, which also seemed to aggravate my insomnia. Then I had my first flare.

This type of flare has nothing to do with sunspots. It's a fibro term used to designate a sudden (or not-so-sudden) exacerbation of symptoms. They aren't the same for everyone, and they aren't always the same each time. We all use different words to describe them, including burning, searing, aching, and cramping. For me, it's as if someone has poured hot oil down my spine. From there, it spreads to my limbs. My neck and back hurt constantly, and the peripheral pain shifts around sporadically and inexplicably. For example, it may start in my lower back and move to my foot to my left arm and back to my calf. If I press on my arm or legs, I can feel tight bands of knotted muscles, sore as hell. Doctors believe increased stress often cause them, but I have kept several diaries and found I seem to be as apt to get a flare when I am on vacation, having a good time, or excited about upcoming plans as I am when I am depressed, disappointed, or overly tired.

As if I couldn't aggravate my condition enough, but still believing that my mental attitude was the biggest contributor to my pain, I decided to take a holiday and drive up to Georgia to visit my oldest son

---

Sleep Hygiene

The following will help you drift off to sleep with or without sleep medications:

Spend the last half hour before bed in a dimly lit room without television

Keep your bedroom cool

Take a hot bath before bed

Drink some herb teas, like chamomile, designed to aid sleep

Eat a small, high-carbohydrate snack

Try to hit the sack at the same time each night

Use your bedroom only for sleeping and sex

If worrying keeps you awake, keep a notepad by your bed and jot down some solutions you can work on the next day

and his family. On the way up, in the middle of what should have been a six- or seven-hour drive, traffic was delayed for three hours because of a fatal traffic accident. When I got to Athens after nearly twelve hours on the road, I could hardly lift my grandchildren. I tried to hide my symptoms from my son and his family. I didn't want them to worry, and I didn't want to ruin our vacation. On the way home, just a few days later, my fingers, wrists, and arms hurt so badly that I could hardly grasp the steering wheel. I considered pulling over and spending the night in a hotel. The only thing that kept me on the road was the fear that I might be getting worse. By the next day, I might not be able to drive at all. I wasn't just driving through northern Florida. I was driving though pain, and I needed to get to the other side as quickly as possible.

Once back in Sarasota, I quickly found a new GP who examined me and ordered routine blood tests. After the blood tests had ruled out thyroid disease, rheumatoid arthritis, lupus, and probably dozens more diseases that I am only vaguely aware of, he was left with one diagnosis: fibromyalgia. I didn't despair. In fact, I was elated to finally have an answer that explained all the strange maladies and lumped them together under one heading.

The doctor had been rather encouraging. He described fibromyalgia as a disease of the nervous system in which neurotransmitters aren't functioning as they should. He said the symptoms had escalated because I had discontinued my antidepressant. I felt assured that I only had to start taking them again and everything would clear up. He also recommended daily workouts. I had always been in pretty good shape, so, despite brutalizing pain, I forced myself through Pilates routines, swimming, walking, running, and tennis.

In the meantime, I sent a résumé to a junior college and immediately found a part-time job teaching English composition. And it looked like the doctor was right. The symptoms did recede for about six weeks. They were a splendid six weeks. I thought I was cured.

I still remember my doctor's beaming smile as I told him about my recovery. He took extra time with me that day. We sat in his office joking and talking about all kinds of things unrelated to my health. Doctors love to help people, and he clearly felt he had helped me.

Then one rainy morning about two months later, I woke up to find all the symptoms had returned. I called the doctor, and he doubled the antidepressant dosage. This happened a couple times. I began to suffer from side effects from the drug, including constipation, lethargy, somnolence, weight gain, loss of sexual interest and, worst of all, increased problems with word recall. Because fibromyalgia and chronic pain can also send you scrambling for a thesaurus to find a word that once was part of your daily vocabulary, it's hard to tell whether it's the drug or the disease. In my case, it's both. I have some problems with word recall even without antidepressants, but the problems increase exponentially when I take the drugs.

My doctor, who had previously been so friendly, now became close-lipped. My visits lasted just a few minutes, long enough for him to write a prescription for a new drug. When I complained about the side effects from the antidepressants, he denied it was the pills and said it was the fibromyalgia. He went on the offensive and began to question me about my lifestyle and my compliance with his suggestions. Was I still exercising? How much did I exercise and for how long? Maybe I needed to get off the couch. He didn't seem to believe me when I told him how much I exercised. Looking back, it seems that, as a doctor, he could have checked my arms, legs, and buttocks for muscle tone, and he would have known I wasn't lying. But he didn't. Once again, it seemed I was doing something wrong and I wasn't fully participating in the doctor's attempt to cure me.

I could hardly talk to him because my mouth was so dry, another side effect of antidepressants. But just saying I had a dry mouth sounds too innocuous. My mouth was bone-dry. My tongue felt like a fallen leaf in November, withered and curled. I could sometimes hardly speak, not a good condition for a teacher. In every class, I kept one or two candied mints in my mouth to keep me salivating. As I looked down at my notes one day, a piece of candy fell out of my mouth and bounced across the room.

"Well, I guess I didn't need that," I said.

The class laughed.

On rare occasions outside of class, I had lost control of my bladder and bowels. I could no longer relax in my classes, fearful I might have a disgusting and very public accident.

I also began to realize that fibromyalgia was a serious diagnosis, not something you recover from with the right prescription and right dose of antidepressants. One of my fellow instructors told me a young female student with fibromyalgia came to class in a wheelchair.

That scared me. I was getting worse every day. I was living with Kevin, but, at that time, there was nothing to stop him from walking out. I was afraid that he didn't realize how serious my illness was and, if he did, he would leave me.

"What if I wind up in a wheelchair?" I asked one day.

"Then I'll just have to learn to push you around," he said casually.

As my health deteriorated,

Is Something Burning?

Just as you wouldn't drive after you've taken a new medication, it's best not to cook either. I once set a dishtowel on fire this way. Every time my husband left for work for weeks after that, he would admonish, "Don't cook! Don't cook! Don't cook!"

I watched him every day, looking for any hint or indication that he wanted me to leave. He owed me nothing. We weren't engaged. Now was the time when he needed to get out. But his love and support stayed strong. He is the most loyal man I have ever known, and I may have never known that if I had not gotten ill. Of course, we were both naïve and optimistic at this point. Over the long term, my illness did take its toll on our relationship in many ways. Although we are still together, it has taken extraordinary effort on both our parts to create a life together. Chronic illness is a chronic stressor on a marriage.

As winter came and I progressively deteriorated, I was on the couch when Kevin left in the morning and on the couch when he returned at night. I got up to teach my classes, but that was all that I could handle. I no longer exercised. I made the effort on occasion, but I was completely wiped out after five minutes.

I was now taking two different kinds of antidepressants, one in the morning and one at night. The second one was supposed to help me sleep. I was sleepy all day, but, every night, I woke up at 1:00 or 2:00 AM, wide-awake. I would lie in bed and listen to the neighbors fighting. The Florida winter fog hung like a curtain between the front walk and me. I was claustrophobic. The humidity overwhelmed me. I had anxiety attacks, among them the fear that I would never sleep again. I would sometimes turn on all the lights in the house, but I still felt lost in the dark.

In the middle of these nights, sleeping in the spare bedroom so as not to disturb Kevin, I read my way through his library. Because he is a big Martin Luther King fan, I became an expert on the civil rights movement. I read books by columnists and about columnists. I read almanacs and grammar guides. I read *A Tale of Two Cities* for the third time. And at 5:00 AM, I would drift off, only to be startled by the alarm clock at 6:00 AM. I stumbled out of bed, groggy and drugged, to teach my 8:00 AM class.

I was pretty good at covering up my mental confusion in class. I pretended it was a game. I adopted the persona of a slightly addled, absentminded professor. After all, professors are supposed to be a bit crazy. When I forgot what I was talking about, I gave them a look of surprise and amusement, as if it were a joke and they were in on it.

"Where were we?" I would ask.

And they would tell me.

"I was just making sure you were paying attention," I said on more than one occasion.

When I was first diagnosed, my doctor never discussed fibro fog with me. I knew I was often disoriented and confused, but I didn't really know it was connected to the fibromyalgia. I often thought it was stress, and I underestimated how muddled my thinking was. But I do know that I misspoke often. I still don't know how many times I might have inadvertently passed something along to my students that was incorrect.

And I felt like hell. I thought I knew what was wrong, lack of sleep and massive doses of antidepressants. But I was starting to learn more about my illness. Now in the middle of the night, I often sat at my computer and typed in the word *fibromyalgia*. I read posts from other patients, checked out chat rooms, and skimmed articles describing symptoms and treatments. I found organizations seeking a cure; medical documents, many on clinical trials of drugs; dozens of professed instant cures; and diagrams of the most common tender points.

So I began to recognize my memory lapses and mental confusion were symptoms, but recognizing that didn't fix them. In fact, memory lapses became more prevalent. The first time I lost my wallet, I left it in a classroom, and the department secretary called me to tell me another teacher turned it in. The second time, I left it in the restroom, and it found its way back to the secretary's office once again. She sounded concerned on the phone and gave me a short lecture. Did I realize all my credit cards were in my wallet? Luckily, no one had taken them, although all my cash was gone the second time.

I lost my wallet again the following week. I had already come home from work when I realized it wasn't there, but I remembered where it was this time. I had put it in my desk drawer in my office. Why I did that, I am not completely sure, but, that night, I drove across town, and I was relieved to find that, at least this time, the secretary wouldn't call me. The fourth time I lost my wallet, someone turned it in to the supervisor of the building, and I was able to get it from him before he returned it to the English department. Once again, my money had disappeared, but the poor students obviously knew better than to try to use someone else's credit cards.

> ### Med Check
> If you are drowsy and don't feel you are on too many drugs already, ask your doctor about Provigil and other medications that can keep you alert and wide-awake.

I no longer lived in a world I could trust. Things seemed to disappear on me, only to turn up somewhere else. I could not remember what I had for breakfast. I often forgot where I was going, even in my own home.

I would start loading the dishwasher and walk into the bathroom to get the cup we used when brushing our teeth. When I got to the bathroom, I would notice the bathroom was dirty and sprinkle cleanser in the sink. Then I would decide to listen to some music while I worked. I would go into the living room, turn on the stereo, and start straightening out a magazine basket.

Only when I picked up a glass that my husband had used to drink his Diet Coke and returned it to the kitchen did I remember that I was loading the dishwasher. Later, when I had to use the bathroom, I would see the cleanser sprinkled in the sink.

I was also in total denial about what was going on. When Kevin noticed how disorganized I was, I blamed him. It was his fault. If he picked up his stuff and put it away, I wouldn't have to.

I thought I was disoriented because, for the first time in years, I was sharing a house with another person. The more frightened I became, the more my denial deepened. I had a list of reasons why I couldn't think straight. I had too much on my mind. Our apartment was so small that I couldn't keep things organized. I was getting old. I had always been this way.[2]

For a woman who used to routinely memorize phone numbers when someone called them out, I found I had to write everything down, including my address and phone number. At odd, unpredictable moments, my mind would go completely blank. I would mentally reach for something, for example, a word to describe the fresh herb I always used in spaghetti, and it was not there. At this stage, I would also sometimes forget what I was reaching for, and I wouldn't remember what the conversation had been about. There were many embarrassing silences where I groped for clues as to what I was expected to say. Two days later, I would remember the correct word, basil.

For the first time, I realized what it was like to have a mental impairment. I now believed in amnesia, something I had always assumed to be a fraud. I was on my way home from school one day when I realized that, although the street looked very familiar, I had no idea where I was. I drove for a couple miles, but nothing improved. I knew I had been on the street, a major thoroughfare, before, even at these intersections, but whether my home was north, south, east, or west, I could not tell you.

I finally pulled over and took out a map, which made no sense to me. I simply sat there for about ten minutes while trying to decide what to do. I knew that more driving would just confuse me. At least this intersection looked familiar.

For no reason that I could explain, the fog in my head finally cleared. I realized I had passed the turnoff to my house by about a mile. I was only a few minutes from home on a five-mile route that I had traveled four times a week for seven months.

By the time the second semester started in January, the antidepressants, even at massive doses and in combinations, were no longer working. My doctor added a new drug, amitriptyline, an antidepressant that also treats insomnia. Within days,

Use It! Don't Lose It!

Keep your mind active, even if it's difficult. Try some of these:

Crossword puzzles

Sudoku

Learning a new language

Jigsaw puzzles

Registering for an online class

---

2   This last excuse was only too true. I had always been something of a space cadet, but now I was a bona fide astronaut.

I had intense nightmares. I woke up screaming in the middle of the night. I didn't always wake up. While I sometimes slept and Kevin sat in the living room watching television, he would hear me moaning or hollering and come to wake me up. They were the kind of nightmares that don't go away when the lights are turned on. I sat in the living room through several nights, staring at the walls while reliving the nightmares, and terrified to go back to sleep because I didn't want to have another one.

I called my doctor and told the nurse the new drug was giving me nightmares.

"How do you know it's the medication?" she asked tartly.

"Because I never have nightmares," I said.

"Well, it looks like you do now."

Neither my doctor nor his nurse wanted to acknowledge the antidepressant's side effects. All my ailments were attributed to the disease. The drugs were infallible. I don't know if the doctors are oversold on the medication by pretty, young drug representatives or if, as a general rule, doctors don't want to discourage patients from trying new drugs. And some of my prescription drugs, Vicodin and Valium, for starters, have had wondrous effects. But I have sometimes had to beg to get them while the doctors liberally disbursed antidepressants, hypertension meds, cholesterol-lowering pills that add to the aches and pains I had, steroids, and a host of others that were also potentially harmful.

Most of the doctors I consulted blanched at the idea of using pain relievers like Vicodin because they believed they were addictive, even though numerous studies have shown that those who use pills for chronic pain and who do not have a history of drug abuse emphatically do not suffer from psychological addiction. Granted, they may suffer physical withdrawal symptoms such as headaches, tremors, or nausea. But even the physical discomfort does not lead to an overwhelming craving for the drug.

On days when my pain level was low, I had no need for them, and I would simply forget to take them. When I smoked cigarettes, I never forgot to smoke. In most cases when I discontinued a drug or switched from one to another, I had no side effects. Now, every week, as my recovery progresses, there are more pain pills left in the plastic oblong container where my pills are sorted into seven separate pockets. Do I crave them? I took OxyContin for several months. When I came off it, I suffered from sweats, nausea, and trembling. But did I want another pill? Certainly not.

Unfortunately, most doctors still believe that everyone who takes painkillers is likely to become psychologically addicted, despite research studies that have shown this is not the case. Srinivasa Raja, professor of anesthesiology at John Hopkins University, found that only 3 percent of chronic pain patients who took pain medication but had no previous history of drug abuse developed psychological dependency to the drugs. The American Pain Society reported his findings in 2008. Chronic pain sufferers like me, who have no past history of drug abuse, do not become addicted because our brains do not associate them with pleasure, only with some relief from pain.

In *The Truth about Chronic Pain*, Arthur Rosenfeld explains the difference between drug tolerance, physical dependence, and addiction. Tolerance is the body's need for an increasing amount of medication to get the same therapeutic effect. Physical dependence occurs when withdrawal of a drug, including cups of coffee, leads to physical symptoms, such as insomnia, nausea, and a host of others. Addiction is something else altogether. It is a biological affliction in which a person has a predisposition to addiction. Pain relievers do not create addicts.

The National Foundation for the Treatment of Pain's Web site backs up this statement with a massive review of research:

State medical boards need to understand that physical dependence and tolerance are not always associated with addiction, thus opiods taken for intractable pain rarely if ever result in addiction.

Unfortunately, doctors are currently regulated by state boards, which keep track of the number of painkillers doctors are prescribing. Doctors don't want to be accused of overprescribing

Getting a Doctor's Attention

Doctors sometimes might be inclined to prescribe the newest medication on the market instead of the tried-and-true one the patient has been taking. To stop this from happening, it might be a good idea to question the doctor about why a certain medicine is better than another and then suggest that you want to check the drug's reliability on the Internet. Hardly any doctor wants to have to refute anonymous comments from the Internet.

narcotics. They also don't want to contribute to pill shoppers like Rush Limbaugh, who visited several doctors with claims of unbearable pain, searching for drugs to feed his addiction to OxyContin.

So GPs often respond to their patients' distress by blithely scribbling script after script for antidepressants, drugs that list six or seven times as many side effects as pain relievers or tranquilizers. It takes months to withdraw from antidepressants with stronger and much more varied and severe withdrawal symptoms than some painkillers.

When I discuss the horrible side effects that antidepressants had on me with doctors, I have been told that I have an unusual response to medication. I sometimes think they are trying to tell me I am mentally unstable. I have had several doctors ask me if I had a psychiatric diagnosis. Did I hear voices? Had I ever been hospitalized for mental illness? Did I or anyone in my family suffer from schizophrenia?

At first, I believed my reactions to the drugs were abnormal. I felt unique. But my responses are no more unique than my fibromyalgia symptoms. If you just type the name of any antidepressant with the word "side effects" into Google, you will find pages and pages of references with hundreds or even thousands of comments from disgruntled users.

I wonder if doctors and their nurses ever read the prescribing information for differing brands of antidepressants, which lists these adverse side effects:

- Coma
- Seizures
- Hallucinations
- Delusions
- Confused states
- Disorientation
- Uncoordination
- Ataxia
- Tremors
- Peripheral neuropathy
- Numbness, tingling, and paresthesias of the extremities

Knowledge Is Power

If you are taking any type of drugs for FMS, you may want to invest in a Physician's Desk Reference (PDR) so you will be fully informed on what you are taking. A PDR will tell you know long the drug has been marketed, how it interacts with other drugs, if it is available as a generic, and even lists other drugs marketed with the same ingredients. A used one can be purchased cheaply at Amazon.com.

- Extrapyramidal symptoms including abnormal involuntary movements and dyskinesia
- Dysarthria
- Disturbed concentration
- Excitement
- Anxiety
- Insomnia
- Restlessness
- Nightmares
- Drowsiness
- Dizziness
- Weakness
- Fatigue
- Headache
- Syndrome of inappropriate ADH (antidiuretic hormone) secretion
- Tinnitus
- Alteration in EEG patterns

When the nurse tried to insist that my nightmares were unrelated to my medication, I didn't buy into it. I never had nightmares. I hadn't since I was a child. I knew this was no fluke. I convinced her to have my doctor change my prescription. He gave me another closely related drug, and the nightmares continued. We tried a third time with Serzone, which gave me terrible headaches. So he added clonazepam, a drug often used to prevent seizures, but also is used as a sedative. This may have improved my sleep by 5 or 10 percent.

In the meantime, the pain began to accelerate. It was soon nearly unbearable. In the middle of the night, I often sat cross-legged in bed, rocking back and forth. I tried adding some over-the-counter medications like aspirin, ibuprofen, and Tylenol, often together. Nothing worked. In desperation, I called a pain clinic and tried to make an appointment. They asked me to have my doctor fax over my medical records, which I did. They called me back to tell me they didn't think there was anything else they could do for me that my doctor wasn't doing.

For several days, I kept hearing that repeatedly in my head, "Nothing we can do for you." I was terrified. What if I never got better? What if I got worse? Exactly what did it mean? Nothing they could do, or nothing anyone could do?

I was afraid to call back and ask them to elaborate. It sounded so final, so hopeless. And the nurse's voice was flat and unsympathetic. I didn't interest them. I didn't qualify as a patient. Were they telling me that my life would become a never-ending nightmare from which there would be no hope of recovery? At that time, I knew very little about chronic pain and the various treatments available.

I am not sure if something in my medical records made them conclude that they couldn't help me or if they simply didn't believe that fibromyalgia was a real disease. Maybe they thought I was looking for narcotics. Actually, maybe I was and didn't know it. I later found the managed use of stronger medicines was a godsend during flares.

Thankfully, not all doctors believe that antidepressants are the only suitable option for FMS. Alina Garcia, a fibromyalgia specialist at the Fibromyalgia and Fatigue Center in Las Vegas, Nevada, explains the process of finding pain relief as a puzzle. "It is like cooking. You can add more salt to the soup ... It's not a linear process. It's more like Sudoku. That's what makes it interesting." Thankfully, as you can see, some doctors out there consider treating fibromyalgia a challenge and intriguing experience rather than a frustration. Dr. Patrick Rhoades, head of the Central Valley Pain Clinic and co-author of this book, is also one of them.

> Doctors see patients with fibromyalgia and they are all depressed. Why are they depressed? Life sucks. At our clinic, when we see patients with fibromyalgia, antidepressants aren't our first drug of choice. We screen for depression before we start writing prescriptions. We do have to consider the side effects of antidepressants. Some patients feel completely numb; they would rather deal with pain than to feel nothing at all. Personally, I prefer to have moments of sadness rather than to feel a hazy kind of happiness all the time. Sometimes patients on antidepressants have emotional reactions that aren't normal. Grieving is normal. Worry is normal. Many times depression is reactive; that is, based

on a divorce or a real problem. I'm not sure antidepressants are the best way to fix that.

Some fibromyalgia patients tend to do very well on
antidepressants. However, the first drug designed specifically for fibromyalgia, Lyrica, doesn't contain an
antidepressant. Not all patients find it effective. Finding
the right pain medication is generally trial and error.

You have to consider each patient as an individual to
find what works for them. Chronic pain management
doesn't have a one-size-fits-all application, but physicians
must take the time to make sure the formula is correct.

But at this point, I was a long way from finding a formula. On
some nights, the pain I suffered was like nothing else I had ever experienced, except perhaps natural childbirth. On these nights, I woke
Kevin up, and he walked the floor with me. He would try to hold me
or pat me, but I couldn't stand the contact. I don't know how many
times I had to ask him not to touch me. That's not easy for a husband
or wife to hear, especially when he or she is trying to soothe a spouse.
It's probably even harder for a boyfriend or girlfriend.

"I just want to die," I told him several times, quietly and earnestly.

He would nod in understanding. I wasn't angry or suicidal in the
clinical way. I couldn't take any more pain. I wasn't trying to run away
from mental problems. I was looking for pain relief. I just didn't want
to hurt anymore.

I realized the doctor, whom I once considered my savior when
he prescribed massive doses of various antidepressants, had no more
answers. Antidepressants were not going to cure me or even bring my
symptoms down to a manageable level. I began to understand that, if
I were ever going to get well, I was going to have to help myself. And
that meant I needed to know more. Much more.

Andrew M., a former electronics technician who also has FMS, says that he and his doctor have been working on finding the right kind of antidepressants: 'one to treat my depression and one that's supposed to help with FM. I take Prozac for depression, and nortriptylin is the one I take for FM. Before bed, I also take two antihistamines. And I take 600 milligrams of guaifenesin twice a day ... this is what I recommend the most.'

Alternative Treatment for Fibromyalgia
& Chronic Fatigue Syndrome

Chapter Four

More Depressing Truths about Antidepressants

"You're on too many meds," said the white-coated young doctor as he looked over my chart. I had recently moved to Modesto, and this was my first visit with him. Then he tried to write me a prescription for nortriptylin, the antidepressant that had given me nightmares a few years before.

"It makes me sick," I protested.

He looked at me skeptically. The medication he wanted me to discontinue was Vicodin.

"Had you ever tried just taking some Motrin? Pain medicines work better if you take less of them," he said. "If you cut out the stronger drugs, Motrin would work just fine."

"How do you feel about Cymbalta (an antidepressant)?"

As usual, he preferred the antidepressant.

"Wonderful drug," he said.

But the pain medicines, those would have to go. Most doctors love antidepressants and for some very good reasons. They have been the wonder drug of the late twentieth century. Before they came along, there was little a family practitioner could do for a depressed patient except recommend a psychiatrist. Now GPs feel qualified to hand them happy pills like candy. They prescribe them for all sorts of reasons. A family practitioner once

Ask Your Pharmacist

If you have a question about your medication and can't reach your doctor, call your pharmacist. He or she can tell you what a safe dose is, what medicines can be taken together, and how long it will take for the drug to wear off.

confided to me that he had put his menopausal wife on antidepressants to make her easier to live with.

"She doesn't like them because she thinks they make her fat," he said with a skeptical look.

I guessed it didn't matter what she thought. After all, he was her doctor and her husband. His admission that he kept his wife on antidepressants sounded disturbingly like a scene out of the *Stepford Wives*.

Have a husband who's unfaithful? Try Zoloft. Your job getting you down? Here's a script for Prozac. Aches and pains? Tired and cranky? Can't sleep? Doctors have been amazed to see their patients coming back a month or two later looking like they had a new lease on life.

So if you want your doctor to think you are truly nuts, just say you don't like antidepressants. Tell him or her that the pills make you emotionally numb, you would like to have an orgasm once in a while, they interfere with your word recall, and they make you feel stupid. Then they will tell you about another one, a brand-new one on the market, that you should try.

I had been convinced, as I pointed out before, that antidepressants would ease the pain and possibly cure my fibromyalgia. Later, as I became better informed, I decided to withdraw from Effexor again. Because I had such horrible side effects the first time I withdrew, I was careful this time to follow the withdrawal schedule the doctor recommended, cutting back to a half-dose for six weeks or so and then stopping them completely. Even then, I started having brain shivers, those electric shocks in the skull, along with headaches, pain spikes, and general malaise. I made my own schedule, gradually reducing them over six months. Interestingly, at this slow pace, the pain did not increase as I withdrew, nor was I more depressed. I doubt I had ever needed Effexor at all.

However, shortly after I had taken my last pill and withdrawn without acute side effects, dizziness overcame me while I was sweeping the floor one day. I fell to my knees and gradually slumped down to the floor. I tried to get up a couple times, but I was much too dizzy. I could feel my heart beating irregularly, something I had never experienced before.

I called to Kevin, who was in the living room. He helped me up and carried me to the couch. As soon as I could sit up comfortably,

I took my pulse. It was skipping every third or fourth beat. It would sometimes skip three or four in a row. I had never in my life felt my heart skip a beat. I thought that was just a hackneyed expression for lovers. Now my heart wasn't just skipping. It seemed like it was stopping. We were both scared.

Kevin drove me to the hospital. The nurse seemed as alarmed as I was, especially when I told her I had no history of any heart disorders. After an EKG, the emergency room doctor told me I was menopausal and stressed. He said I probably had always had an arrhythmia all my life. It had just become more pronounced. It was certainly an amazing diagnosis. I couldn't imagine how this arrhythmia could have gone unnoticed by dozens of doctors, nurses, and other medical professionals throughout my whole life. And how had I never noticed it, all the years when I took my pulse twice in every aerobics class at least three times a week? He shrugged. As far as he was concerned, I was fine. My blood pressure was only slightly elevated, and I wasn't dying.

Two days later, I called the only doctor I knew personally, an emergency room doctor I had once dated. I asked him how an arrhythmia could go undetected for fifty-four years. He suggested I might have ventricular premature complexes, a disorder common to high-strung women, and suggested I follow up with my family doctor. My family doctor ordered a stress test, which I passed even though I can't describe how painful it was for me to jog. The doctors weren't concerned. My blood pressure was 120/90. I had no shortness of breath. Their indifference scared me. Call me an idiot, but having a heart that skips every third or fourth beat can't be good for you, especially if you plan on living for another thirty years or so. It was particularly frightening during my habitual middle-of-the-night anxiety attacks when I would lie awake, checking my pulse over and over as it skipped and skipped and skipped. Never once during that time did my heart make it to thirty beats without at least one skip. It sometimes skipped as many as six or seven beats in a row.

I asked my family doctor the same question I had asked both emergency room doctors. Could the arrhythmia be related to my withdrawal from Effexor? All three emphatically said no.

However, as early as 2000, the *Medicine Herald* published an article by two Chinese scientists, Su Qiaorong and Sun Shouqing, with conclusive evidence that arrhythmia was one of the dozens of side effects of antidepressant withdrawal syndrome, as it is now called by drug companies. How did doctors miss compelling evidence about antidepressant withdrawal for so long? Ever notice those good-looking, personable, overdressed individuals with briefcases in your doctor's office who don't look sick enough to be there? These are drug reps, and they make impressive salaries by peddling their wares to your doctor. My daughter-in-law, a beautiful, blonde, former college cheerleader, used to be one of them. She is not an anomaly. On November 28, 2005, the *New York Times* published an article by Stephanie Saul about how drug companies were using sex to sell drugs. Many of the sales representatives are former cheerleaders. Here is an excerpt:

> Anyone who has seen the parade of sales representatives through a doctor's waiting room has probably noticed that they are frequently female and invariably good looking. Less recognized is the fact that a good many are recruited from the cheerleading ranks.

Cheerleading ranks? You betcha. Sales recruiters say cheerleaders have persuasive enthusiasm that carries over to pharmaceutical sales. Never mind that they are also beautiful, physically fit, and overwhelmingly female while most doctors are overwhelmingly male.

One of the Washington Redskins cheerleaders earned her living at a nine-to-five job, counseling doctors on the advantages of a treatment for vaginal yeast infections.

The article also quotes Dr. Thomas Carli of the University of Michigan, "There's a saying that you'll never meet an ugly drug rep."

Former cheerleaders do not need a degree in biology or chemistry. They need a toothpaste smile and exaggerated enthusiasm. There are no statistics on how many of the nation's ninety thousand drug reps are former cheerleaders, but there is enough demand that some individuals have established personnel firms just to recruit cheerleaders into the pharmaceutical ranks, where starting salaries begin at as much as $50,000 to $60,000 a year and quickly ease up to six figures. The job market for former cheerleaders is so strong that George C. Webb founded Spirited Sales, a job placement firm, in the early 1990s, specifically to recruit cheerleaders and place them in jobs with sales organizations. On his Web site, www.spiritedsales.com, he asks:

> Are you interested in making yourself available to an exciting career in medical sales? Do you have the experience of performing in front of thousands of people and representing your institution to students, faculty and alumni?

His company, which has recently expanded to include other types of athletes, dancers, and college leaders, helps applicants with their résumés and charges a one-time fee of $2,500 if the prospective employee is placed in an organization. He promises to arrange interviews with leading pharmaceutical companies and help them prepare for the interview. Webb also told the *Times*:

> The cheerleaders now are the top people in universities; these are really capable and high-profile people. There's a lot of sizzle in it. I've had people who are going right out, maybe they've been out of school for a year, and get a car and make up to $50,000, $60,000 with bonuses, if they do well.

Of course, not all antidepressants are sold by cheerleaders, and not all former cheerleaders sell antidepressants. And the cheerleaders do receive company training on the medications they sell. But doctors are only human. If pretty, young females couldn't more easily sway them, the marketing departments of major pharmaceutical companies would know about it. Then the sweet young things who majored in physical education would be replaced by geeky-looking biochemistry majors, if doctors preferred them.

Another sales technique used by drug salesmen is the free lunch. I was standing at the desk signing in for an appointment once as a drug representative tried to talk his way into a meeting with the doctor. The busy nurse rebuffed him.

"Can I set up a lunch?" he asked.

The receptionist looked up and said to me, "I don't need any more information from you. You can sit down."

But I kept standing as she agreed that he could indeed set up a lunch. It seems she didn't even need to consult the doctor for this. From under the desk, she pulled out a calendar, obviously kept just for that purpose.

"How about the twenty-eighth?" she asked.

He agreed and handed her his card. She wrote the date in a calendar book.

"How many on your staff?" he asked.

"About fifteen," she said.

"Around noon?" he asked.

She nodded.

"Any kind of food you particularly like?" he asked.

She glanced at me. We both knew I was eavesdropping with interest.

"No," she said.

"Twelve it is then," he said, picking up his briefcase gingerly and heading for the door.

To be fair, other factors besides free lunches and pretty cheerleaders push doctors toward prescribing antidepressants for fibromyalgia patients. As I said earlier, in most doctors' experience and in clinical trials, the antidepressants and other drugs seem to work. Of course, the tests don't last for months or years. For fibromyalgia, antidepressants do seem to improve symptoms, at least at first. After a while, of course, the benefits wear off, and the doses have to be increased, and withdrawal symptoms are painful. And the withdrawal symptoms are often attributed to a flare-up of symptoms, adding to the doctor's conviction that the antidepressants were keeping the condition under control.

There's another reason doctors tend to prescribe antidepressants for fibromyalgia that has nothing to do with pretty girls. They simply don't know much about FMS. Many doctors who completed their medical training before 1995 were taught that fibromyalgia was a psychological disorder. Unfortunately, many doctors don't keep up with the latest scientific literature for most diseases, not just fibromyalgia. So when a drug rep comes in with the latest medication proven to be effective, it's an easy answer.

Many doctors receive credit for continuing education courses taught by drug representatives. Dr. Alina Garcia, the fibromyalgia expert in Las Vegas, said that, after medical school, many doctors receive most of their ongoing training from drug representatives. Certainly, no one would disagree that doctors must keep abreast of the latest information on new drugs, but one could argue that drug manufacturers are least likely to be objective about their products.

Also, in some cases, there is financial incentive. My daughter-in-law told me that the most frequent questions doctors asked was how the stock of a particular drug company was doing. No law prevents doctors from investing in drug companies and reaping the benefits when the stocks from companies that produce the drugs they prescribe go up. They are also the first to know when a new drug is coming along that might affect a drug company's Wall Street performance. But even doctors who have no financial incentives peevishly defend their favorite drugs and brush off complaints of side effects. Most don't like to admit they were wrong. If doctors sometimes appear to be godlike, it may be because they have to play god every day. One wrong decision, one dead patient.

It should make them cautious. Instead, it often makes them imperious. They have to believe in themselves, sometimes in the face of overwhelming disasters. As a former newspaper editor, I had to make instant decisions every day. Some were mistakes. The worst that could happen with me was that someone's reputation might be tarnished. We could get sued. Certainly, I might be publicly embarrassed. But no one died.

You would think the life-and-death responsibility would motivate doctors to slow down, see fewer patients, read charts carefully, and spend more time with patients. But in our profit-driven medical system, doctors too often grope for quick answers and one-size-fits-all solutions. Not only do they dislike it when you argue with them because it hurts their ego, they don't have time for it.

It takes less time to write a prescription, and it's relatively safe. Even if early drug trials sufficient to get the drug on the market don't always uncover long-term problems, most of the drugs aren't deadly at first.

So the doctor prescribes medication, and it often works for a while. Then the patient deteriorates again. It's likely that the doctor interprets this, not as a failure of the drug, but as a worsening of the patient's disease. Then another drug rep comes in with a new, improved antidepressant that is more effective than the last, and the doctor switches his or her patients to the new one. And the cycle begins again.

One of these new, improved antidepressants is Cymbalta. After one particularly bad flare, in sheer desperation, I was talked into trying it because, as I was told, it was "the best thing there was for chronic pain." And it may well be. I know Cymbalta reduced my pain, but, like all the other antidepressants, it made me feel strange. The doctors insisted that, if I took it for a few months, the side effects would diminish. And they did. So I continued them. Naturally, they had to increase my dosage eventually, and there were more side effects to adjust to. But I took them because I was in so much pain that I would have taken anything that might help, even if it meant taking years off my life. If you haven't had this kind of pain before, think of childbirth, passing a kidney stone, or a migraine. Think about worrying, as your sleeping pill knocks you out, that tomorrow might be worse and wishing you wouldn't wake up.

So I took them for months, knowing I would not be able to discontinue them until I was stable and vastly improved. After eight months, I told my GP I wanted to quit taking them.

"Well, I guess you could," he said.

"Well, I'm not sure they're helping anymore," I said. "Don't you want me to stop taking any drugs that I don't need to take?"

He shrugged and then cautioned me about weaning off the pills gradually. He suggested I drop from sixty milligrams to thirty and then discontinue them completely in three weeks. I told him I had problems when I quit taking Effexor, everything from insomnia to arrhythmia, and how I had ended up at the emergency room.

"This isn't the same as Effexor. You shouldn't have problems with this," he said.

"You don't seem like you think this is a good idea," I said.

"I just don't know why anyone would want to stop taking Cymbalta," he said.

"Why not?"

"Because I think it's a wonderful drug," he said.

This doctor had told me I was overmedicated and said I didn't need Vicodin and Valium. But he was enamored with Cymbalta, which has an even longer list of side effects and precautions. In addition, Cymbalta had only been on the market for a couple of years, so its side effects, especially the complications of withdrawal, were not yet completely understood. Before I started to decrease my pills, I intended to do some research on withdrawing from Cymbalta. I didn't want to have the same problems I had when I was withdrawing from Effexor. It seemed pretty straightforward at the time.

I cut back to half the dosage for about a week without any problem. Then I started throwing up and feeling weak and dizzy, and the pain level shot up from a five to an eight. Obviously, I had cut down too fast. I started taking a full dose one day and a half-dose the next for a week. Then, once again, I tried to cut down to thirty milligrams every day.

Meantime, at night, I got on the Internet and typed in "Cymbalta withdrawal." Hundreds of Web sites came up. Near the top of the first page was a site called "Cymbalta hell." Hundreds, maybe thousands, of fellow sufferers had left messages on numerous chat boards, detailing dozens of side effects, some deadly serious. Many had made visits to the emergency room. A few mentioned lawsuits. So, while I knew I might have trouble discontinuing it, I vastly underestimated the difficulty.

Cymbalta is a long-lasting drug. It builds up in your bloodstream over days instead of hours, so, the first few days after I had cut my dosage in half, I had enough in my system to still feel pretty good.

The worst symptoms didn't begin until the following week. The first thing I noticed was that the sun seemed too bright. The slightest noise seemed painful. Like many others with chronic pain, I am sensitive to the faintest odors. Because we lived in farm county, I smelled the manure, cows, and turkey farms. And I vomited. I shook. I sweated. The pain soared. I was too dizzy to get up, and it was too painful to lie down. I suffered from bad dreams, perhaps not nightmares, but dreams too vivid to disappear when the bedroom light came on. It was like a bad case of the flu, but worse because the symptoms were so much more disconcerting and frightening. I felt like I had woken up in outer space. Absolutely nothing, not even the pictures of my children, looked familiar. It was the worst and longest-lasting panic attack I have ever had.

I suffered through a week of this, and then the symptoms subsided. Somewhat recklessly, but eager to get off a drug I now saw as deadly, I quit taking it completely. Within a few days, the withdrawal symptoms returned in a much higher resonance. The pain that was disabling two weeks ago was now unbearable. I lived in a universe that I can only describe as unreal, harsh, and glaring, where everything was too bright, hot, loud, and vivid. I was swimming on a hot summer day with the sun burning down on the cool water. I had this sense that I was alone in the universe, on a wavelength that was both too short and too long to allow me to communicate with Kevin, my friends, my children, and even my pets. Sunshine hurt; trees hurt. I had no love or compassion for anyone, only a weak desire to try to find my way back, if I knew where to go.

I wondered if this was what psychosis felt like. I understood why so many of the mentally ill kill themselves. I did not fear death as much as another day in the overwhelming mental and physical agony. Then the physical pain shot up. Obviously, the antidepressants had been controlling my pain whether I wanted to admit it or not. Late on a Friday afternoon, too late to reach my doctor, the pain finally reached a ten on a scale of ten. I paced the living room floor, as I had done in childbirth. I thought about driving to the emergency room, but I wasn't sure I could make it. I also considered calling Kevin and asking him to come home from work, but, because the pain level so often rose and fell, I was afraid I would be better before he got there.

Feeling desperately alone, I called my sister Darlene, who also suffers from fibromyalgia, but I hurt too much to talk. At first, she tried asking me questions, but, getting nowhere, she finally asked, "What if I just talk to you to try to keep your mind off the pain?"

For hours, I listened to the comforting music of my sister's voice as she talked about our sisters and brothers, her children, and God knows what else. It reminded me of the time I had been sick in Florida, and Kevin had read to me. I don't remember much of what she said that day, but every word helped ease the pain. Every sentence reminded me that there was a life beyond all this and that, if I could just hang on, I could get back there … maybe.

On Saturday, I was a bit better. By Sunday afternoon, I was vomiting and walking the floor again. Kevin was off work that day, and he tried to help by massaging me, but, by 5:00 PM, there was no way out. I had to go to the emergency room.

When we arrived at dinnertime on that hot Sunday afternoon, the waiting room was crowded and dirty. At least thirty patients were ahead of me, some in wheelchairs and most in obvious despair. I walked the floor, sometimes indoors and sometimes outside, where smokers in wheelchairs enjoyed their cigarettes. After an hour or two, a nurse called me in to take my medical history. The nurse knew nothing about Cymbalta withdrawal. It was obvious she didn't believe a word I was saying about it. When I mentioned that I had read about dozens of other cases just like this on the Internet, she put her hand on my arm.

"Leave the Internet alone," she said. "That kind of thing just gets you going. You have to just trust your doctor."

Finally, at my insistence, she asked me to spell the name of the drug that I blamed for my withdrawal symptoms, but I could tell she had no confidence in what I was telling her.

"Have you always had high blood pressure?" she asked casually.

"How high is her blood pressure?" Kevin asked.

"210/120," she said.

Kevin gasped.

"I don't have high blood pressure," I said.

"You do now," she replied curtly.

"But that's because I'm in pain," I said.

She gave me a skeptical look, but then resumed her professional look-I-really-care-but-I'm-really-busy smile.

"We'll get you feeling better soon," she said confidently as we left to return to the waiting room. I wondered at her confidence. No one had been able to "get me feeling better soon" in ten years, but this emergency room was going to do it as soon as they could get to me.

"We'll call you right away," she added.

But they didn't do that either. From the looks on the worn faces on the number of patients who had been there longer than I had been, I knew they wouldn't. They were averaging

One at a Time

Occasionally FMS patients who are fed up with their medications because of side effects or because they feel the medication isn't effective will stop taking all their medications at once. This is potentially very dangerous. Always consult your doctor before discontinuing your medication so that he can monitor it.

four or five patients an hour. At this rate, I could have been there until midnight.

About 9:00 PM, about three hours after we arrived, I started to feel just a bit better. It was also time to take my sleeping pill. While I debated whether to go home, try to knock myself out, and go to the doctor's office the next day, I went in to use the restroom, which was near the door to the emergency room.

I have only smelled death a few times in my life, once when I went in to see my father just a few minutes after he had been pronounced dead, but I never forgot that sweet, sickly smell. And I could smell death emanating from the emergency room. I suppose a doctor might say that also was just a hallucination that the intractable pain brought on, but I doubt it. It was enough to send me home, thankful some overworked and uninformed intern hadn't gotten the opportunity to make a bad choice and give me a painkiller that, given the imbalance that my body was in due to the withdrawal, would be fatal.

Kevin was only too happy to get me out of there. He fed me, gave me my meds, and put me to bed. The first medication I took was a full dose, sixty milligrams of Cymbalta. I couldn't fight these effects of withdrawal anymore.

The next day, my family physician, the one who had extolled the benefits of Cymbalta and told me I would have "no problem" getting off it, listened impassively as I explained my failed attempt at withdrawal. A few months ago, he said I could withdraw safely in a matter of weeks, but, when I told him about my aborted trip to the emergency room, he admitted that 20 percent of patients who try to withdraw from the drug end up with antidepressant discontinuation syndrome, a serious condition that can lead to psychosis.

"Will I ever get off Cymbalta?" I asked.

"Well, not for at least a year," he said.

I balked at that.

"Well, I wouldn't try again for at least six months," he said.

So I would continue indefinitely to suffer from the side effects, headaches, dizziness, problems with word recall (a serious problem for a writer), and constipation. I would later withdraw from OxyContin with much less discomfort. In the meantime, to this day, I am dependent on Cymbalta.

But, as I discovered from the Internet, I am one of the more fortunate ones. As much as I disliked restarting Cymbalta, I could afford to take it. My insurance covered it, and the doctor's office was happy to provide me with free samples. The Internet is full of stories of patients who had to stop Cymbalta because patients could no longer afford it. The cost of the drug, without insurance, is roughly $200 monthly. Yet never once, in the ten or fifteen times antidepressants have been prescribed for me, was I ever told about the painful and even dangerous withdrawal, nor did it appear on the information sheet that comes with the drug. What's more, no pharmacist ever told me what to expect. Only recently has a disclaimer been added to the Cymbalta prescribing information fact sheet your pharmacist will give you with the drug. It reads:

> During marketing of SSRIs and SNRIs (serotonin and norephinephrine reuptake inhibitors), there have been spontaneous reports of adverse events occurring upon discontinuation of these drugs, particularly when abrupt, including the following: dysphonic mood, irritability, agitation, sensory disturbances (e.g., paresthesias such as electric shock sensations), anxiety, confusion, headache, lethargy, emotional lability, insomnia, hypomania, tinitus, and seizures. Although these events are self-limiting, some have been reported to be severe.

Can't Afford Your Meds?

Let your doctor know right away. He may be able to keep you supplied with free samples handed out by drug sales representatives. Some pharmaceutical companies also have special programs in which they provide prescription drugs for low-income patients. You may also be able to switch to a low-cost generic.

This has a very different tone than the user-friendly guide on Cymbalta's Web site, where it answers users' questions, such as "What happens when I stop taking Cymbalta?" It reads:

> Like other antidepressants, Cymbalta should not be stopped suddenly. Stopping Cymbalta suddenly may

> result in symptoms like dizziness, nausea or head-
> ache. Talk with your doctor or healthcare professional
> before stopping Cymbalta as he or she may wish to
> decrease the dose slowly to help you avoid these kinds
> of symptoms.

No mention of intolerable symptoms like dysphonic mood, which is roughly defined as feelings of guilt, anxiety, and depression; electric shock sensations; emotional lability, a medical term for heightened emotional responses; or stroke. Antidepressants may also cause tardive dyskinesthesia, or involuntary movement. I have it in my right hand, which often moves of its own accord.

To be fair, many people, including me, have been helped by the use of antidepressants and other pain medication, and I believe in these drugs. They can sometimes be lifesaving by relieving intractable pain. But, if I had been told about the difficulties of withdrawal, I undoubtedly would have tried other medications first and would only have taken it as a last resort.

Perhaps doctors feel patients might be reluctant to try new drugs if they are fully informed about the side effects. Maybe they are just too busy to answer questions. But how could a drug like Cymbalta be marketed and prescribed before doctors and patients were informed of the side effects of withdrawal? Did the drug companies know about this? Were doctors informed?

What is worse, at the same time, most traditional doctors will refuse to prescribe painkillers like Percocet or Ultram. If they do, they will be lecturing you about the dangers of addiction. I have never had a bit of trouble withdrawing from painkillers after the pain has diminished. And these drugs have been on the market so long that a plethora of generic versions are available. They are not terribly profitable for drug companies. Sadly, most doctors don't listen to their patients. They listen to their drug reps. So, while most FMS patients have been frightened away from painkillers by their doctors, they are taking drugs that may not be psychologically addictive, but have extremely painful withdrawal from the physical addiction. Of course, doctors prefer to call it "withdrawal syndrome" rather than addiction.

So my doctor, who steadfastly objected to the use of painkillers or sedatives like Vicodin and Valium, which I could quit taking at any time without side effects, had no qualms about pushing Cymbalta on his patients as an alternative for pain relief and its companion, depression.

I wish I could have dealt with chronic pain without ever taking antidepressants or pain relievers, but prescribed drugs are still the best treatment I have found. However, once you begin to take these drugs, it's in your best interest to find a doctor who specializes in pain relief. Because these medications are serious, you want a doctor with vast experience in prescribing them, one who will know what to watch for while he or she is treating you. Having a pain specialist prescribe all your medication also makes it less likely that your doctors will prescribe medications that should not be taken together.

Cymbalta and other antidepressants can be extremely effective. They may have saved my life during the darkest days of my suffering. But we live in times when drugs have become extremely complicated, and all of us react to drugs differently. You are the expert on your own body, and being aware of potential side effects and withdrawal syndromes can save you a great deal of stress when you experience strange physical and mental conditions.

Imagine yourself free from the complex symptoms of Chronic Fatigue and Fibromyalgia. Imagine how you will feel if you didn't have to worry about it ever again or have to deal with the negative side effects of any pharmaceutical drugs. Well, it's not just a dream ... it can be a reality.

Ad taken from Web site advertising
a nutritional ad

Chapter Five

The Predators of Positive Thinking

The nutritional supplement guaranteed to cure me came in the mail, $120 for a four-week supply. It was another addition to my credit card bill. It was a powder and might have been of more use if I had mixed it into a paste and used it to seal envelopes. But, if I had to do it over again, would I have ordered it? Probably. I was desperate. If the cost is reasonable and a vitamin formula or herbal supplement is safe, I don't think there's any harm in trying it. Some FMS sufferers claim they have improved with some of these products, especially glucosamine sulfate. As for vitamins, each one of us has different nutritional needs, and you certainly want to make sure you have enough calcium, magnesium, zinc, and other essential vitamins and minerals. But be careful. You can overdose on some vitamins, and amino acids and other miracle cures can cause more havoc with your system.

Besides the herbal and diet supplements, I spent a chunk of my dwindling savings on fibromyalgia books. I found dozens, if not hundreds, of suggestions. I felt empowered. The books assured me I could reverse, control, and relieve my condition. But they generally failed me in the end. Some things reduced my pain; some gave me temporary relief. But, without a competent medical professional to guide me through them and make sure I had appropriate tests and evaluations, they weren't as effective as they should have been.

Worse, after reading some of the hard-core you-have-to-think-positive-or-you'll-never-improve FMS literature, I felt like a failure when I didn't improve. If I didn't follow through on every suggestion or I cheated and ate a piece of cheesecake after being told that sugar was the root of all my problems, I blamed myself. I think these books should come with a disclaimer, "Here are some suggestions, but, if they don't work, it's not your fault."

There are a few Web sites where you will find treatments for fibromyalgia and other illnesses ranked for their effectiveness by patients like you and me. Some of the most effective treatments are comfortable mattresses, at 87 percent, followed by rest at 81 percent. Of course, your doctor probably won't prescribe either of these, and you won't read about them in most fibromyalgia survival books. Mattress sellers obviously haven't learned to market their product to doctors. GPs tend to stick to generally practical prescriptions, like antidepressants, Motrin, and exercise.

Among other treatment I tried were magnets, which were listed at one of these Web sites as effective for 66 percent of patients. They were cheaper than the nutritional supplements. You can get them in the form of bracelets, belt buckles, or tiny ones shaped like coins that you tape all over your body. Overall, they didn't work for me, although I have heard others who swear by them. But I do suspect that I benefited from a placebo effect. For the first few days, the magnets seemed to pull the pain right out of me. I danced. I cleaned the house. I walked briskly and gleefully from the classroom where I taught to my office. I was amazed. I hadn't believed that magnets would work! That lasted about a week. Then whatever magic they had was gone. I've heard this story over and over again from fibromyalgia patients about various treatments. "It seemed to work for awhile, but then ..."

What we as patients often don't take into account is spontaneous remission. Fibromyalgia symptoms fluctuate on a daily, weekly, monthly, or even hourly basis. So when I slapped on those magnets, I was pretty likely heading into remission at the same time.

"Wow," I thought, "these gadgets really work."

But when I felt lousy again the next week, I ripped them off and threw them in the garbage. Perhaps magnets work for some of us, but not others. Because magnets are inexpensive and won't hurt you, they are worth trying.

I may have been experiencing the placebo effect with magnets. There are two ways to consider placebos:

• Placebos support the theory that you can get well if you believe you can. All you have to do is keep a positive attitude. I wish it were that simple. Positive thinking is clearly good medicine. It will relax you and help you deal with your pain. Perhaps it will even diminish it. Positive thinking may help if you are hovering between illness and wellness. It may tip you over to the wellness side. But it's tough to fix a broken leg or serious physical problem with faith alone. Fibromyalgia is some sort of physical abnormality. The abnormally high levels of Substance P in the spinal column in FMS patients have been documented. Substance P is a protein that functions as a neurotransmitter, and its function is to excite the nerves in cases where patients suffer from arthritis or low back pain.

• Some patients may have a positive attitude because they can sense that their body is up to the task of recovery. After all, your body belongs to you. Generally, if you are recovering from a cold or the flu, you are the first to know. And you don't need a doctor to tell you. Could a positive attitude result from the body's ability to evaluate its own strength in overcoming an illness? The brain and the body, working together, sense the patient has enough strength to overcome his or her physical ailment, and this is responsible for the so-called positive attitude that some physicians and faith healers believe can cure illness. Or maybe, in the case of patients who don't recover, the body has already sent a subtle signal that says, "There's no way you are going to overcome this." The patient is gloomy; the doctor blames the patient. But would a doctor blame a patient for a burst appendix? It seems the patient gets the blame when there is nothing more the doctor can do. The doctor and a positive attitude get the credit for recovery.

In *Running on Empty*, Katrina Berne, a clinical psychologist, summarizes the problems with modern medicine:

When physicians lack a biomedical model that explains patient complaints, they revert to psychiatric diagnoses:

Fact or Myth?

Much of the literature on fibromyalgia insists that FMS patients are overachievers. While this could be true, it's also likely that, when doctors first see the patients, they are already overwhelmed and unable to keep up with their activities. They may look and feel frazzled and frantic, even if they had never been that way before their illness.

---

depression, somatization disorder, or malingering. They are trained to cure people and that's what they like to do. When they can't fix what's wrong, they become frustrated, their professional identities threatened. We don't get better, and we don't go away. We just keep coming back with the same complaints and additional new ones.

There is this insanity in American medicine that patients are to blame for whatever doctors can't cure. It's a variation on the theme of faith healing, only we no longer rely on strangers to put their hands on our heads and help us walk again.

"You have to keep a positive attitude," doctors have told me at times when I could barely walk because of the crippling pain. Like if I would just cheer up, I would be signing up for a marathon in a few weeks. At first, I really did feel as if I were to blame for my lack of progress. Then I got mad ... really mad. And every fibromyalgia patient I have ever talked to has blamed herself or himself for the lack of progress at some point.

Don't get me wrong. As I said, I prefer to have a positive attitude, and I do think a positive attitude may have an effect on your well-being and even perhaps on reducing your pain and other symptoms. But if you could cure diseases with positive attitudes, there would be no use for doctors. When you have an accident and break a leg, no one says to you, "Well, you're not going to get well if you don't have a positive attitude." Doctors splint your leg, tell you not to reinjure it, and give you pain meds. When you have a certified real condition, they don't lecture you about how you are sabotaging your progress.

Ironically, while doctors rely on positive thinking from the placebo effect to cure something that they can't, they will completely dismiss most alternative therapies, like magnets, vitamin therapies, and even acupuncture as bogus, even though it's clear that many of these therapies, even if they fail to prove themselves effective in clinical trials, often give patients the positive thinking that the doctors want so badly to see.

Researchers have enough evidence to prove that the placebo effect does work, at least for a small percentage of the population. And while researchers may hate it because it complicates the statistics when they conduct drug research and other treatment effectiveness trials, it's confusing when doctors want you to have a positive attitude, but don't want you to attribute improvement to anything other than their own solicitous care. Traditional Western doctors don't want you to believe in colon cleansing, ginseng, raw food diets, or other treatments, but they want you to believe you will get better, even when you are screaming from bad dreams at night and tormented with searing pain by day.

Thankfully, some more enlightened doctors are moving away from blaming patients with diseases that are not well understood. Some recommend therapies today that were unheard of a few decades ago, including Tai Chi, massage, acupuncture, and even magnets. There are many doctors with more enlightened attitudes.

But no one really knows enough to claim that upbeat attitudes can cure physical diseases, although clinical trials and other evidence points to some kind of interaction between emotional states and wellness.

Some early studies suggested that patients who had someone pray for them improved at a higher rate than other patients, even when the patients didn't know the individuals who prayed for them. But the largest, best-funded study, conducted at Templeton University, disproved the theory.

In 2006, the *Boston Globe* reported that Templeton University had conducted a study in which 1,802 bypass patients were divided into two groups. The members of one group were assigned someone to pray for them, unknown to the patient. The $2.4 million study failed to find any difference in the outcome of the two groups of patients.

There are case histories of patients with terminal cancer who vowed to cure themselves and did. But, for every anecdote of survival, there are a hundred stories where the patients died.

Sure, it's better to think positive. It's certainly more pleasant to have hope. But, in my case, I think I can prove that positive thinking hurt me more than helped by encouraging me to do things I wasn't capable of. And my doctors helped me hurt myself.

So if today is a day when you just can't summon up one positive thought, don't blame yourself. We all have days like that, sometimes lots of them. The best thing you can do on a day like that is call a friend, preferably another fibromyalgia patient, and get a huge dose of understanding.

A disease presents itself in a unique form in each person it attacks, and it pursues a unique course. A good or bad prognosis is a statement of probability, not of fact. Every individual responds to treatment differently than any other.

Sherwin B. Nuland, *The Wisdom of the Body*

Chapter Six

Alternatives

Having warned against snake oil medicine, medical practitioners, and others who seem to think you can cure yourself if you would just get happy, I want to emphasize that many alternative treatments are worth trying and many of them bring relief, albeit often temporary.

I think many of these improve your overall health. Whatever you can do to keep yourself healthy will help with any syndrome or disease, not just FMS. If you find some alternatives look interesting, you can afford them, and they have no adverse side effects, why not try them? To me, taking action is an act of faith and a more effective one than sitting around depressed because I can't cure myself with happy thoughts.

Chinese and other Asian remedies have been godsends for me, particularly acupuncture. The first year after I was diagnosed, acupuncture provided the greatest relief. I literally counted the hours until my next acupuncture appointment. A single treatment didn't completely stop the pain, but it did bring it down to a manageable level. Often, as I walked the floor in the middle of the night, I dreamed they would someday have emergency clinics for acupuncture that would be open all night. Maybe they will someday.

I tried acupuncture for the first time after I found an article on the Internet that said that 70 percent of fibromyalgia patients improved with acupuncture. I am not sure where I found the article or if those

---

A Doctor Confesses

A neurosurgeon once told me he had used magnets on his belt for years to control his back pain while he was performing surgery. He said he didn't know how they worked, but they did. And who recommended them to him? An anesthesiologist, who noticed he was stooped over and stiff during operations.

---

figures still hold up because I don't know if they came from a reputable source. I wasn't thrilled about getting stuck with needles all over my already painfully sore body, but the avowed 70 percent success rate was better than anything else I had read about.

With some apprehension, I visited a thin, energetic young doctor of Oriental medicine who had trained in China. He wasn't interested in what Western doctors said about my fibromyalgia. Instead, he looked in my throat and ears and listened to my pulse.

"Pain is a condition that is filled with many things," he said mysteriously.

In his diagnosis, my body was filled with infection that had become stagnant. In other words, my Chi wasn't moving. I had a yin imbalance. It took months of studying the basics of Chinese medicine before his words made any sense to me.

I felt some relief from the acupuncture, but it didn't last more than a few hours at first. Then, as I returned for treatments three times a week for several weeks, I improved.

Homeopathy

This is a theory that substances that cause adverse effects, such as allergies, can be used to cure small doses of the offending substance.

It is a hotly debated, but highly popular, remedy.

I told him I exercised faithfully every day, and he told me to stop it immediately and just rest. Rest is the top-rated remedy when fibromyalgia patients rate their own treatments online, but every conventional Western doctor I have ever visited has always told me to step up the exercise. After all, many of us are overweight. Western doctors tend to think we are slugs, couch potatoes to such a degree that we are soft and sprouting. But when you think about how most of us live, balancing families, careers, friends, foes, and bill collectors, it's much more likely that we are exhausted.

The acupuncturist told me to get out in the sunshine and just sit.

"You are much too weak," he said. He also said he could tell I was the type of person who was "always busy, too busy," he said in his limited English. It was time to "not be too busy."

Of course, I thought he was crazy at first. How could so many American doctors be wrong? But I finally gave in and stopped struggling through those excruciating workouts that left me hurting more than before. He also gave me foul-tasting herbs and told me to give up sugar and eat only fresh foods.

After three weeks or so, my pain level went down from an eight or nine to a six or seven. I could always count on the acupuncture to bring my pain down a notch or two. I had finally found a reliable treatment.

Once I started my acupuncture and my symptoms began to recede, I tried to discontinue my antidepressant once more. The acupuncture didn't stop withdrawal from setting in. My pain level soared, the brain zaps returned, and I couldn't sleep. My acupuncturist surprised me by telling me to start taking the drugs again, at least until I was well on my way to getting better.

"Right now your body needs them," he said.

I read more books on acupuncture and Eastern medicine and discovered an entirely different perspective on health. Most Western doctors look for the one-size-fits-all treatment. If a doctor sees a patient with arthritis, the prescribed therapy is always the same: the same drugs, physical therapy, or perhaps a joint replacement or other surgery, depending on the location of the arthritis.

A Chinese doctor might prescribe completely different treatments. He may treat one patient for Chi deficiency and another for congealed blood, all conditions unrecognized by Western medicine. The Eastern doctor looks beyond the disease to the entire biological system. To an acupuncturist, disease occurs when the body is out of balance. A healthy body can ward off illness, which explains why some of us get colds and others don't. In ancient China, if a patient became ill under an acupuncturist's care, the patient didn't have to pay because the doctor had obviously failed. Patients sought medical care not when they

---

Nothing but the Best ...

If you are willing to try everything and have an unlimited budget, a health center that treats fibromyalgia, located in lovely and wholesome southern Utah, offers a nineteen-day retreat, complete with Western physicians, psychologists, chiropractors, acupuncturists, massage, pool, therapy, yoga, and even a Native American healer for $17,900, unless your insurance will help. In which case, it will only cost you $9,900. For this, you share a room with two others. If you can't afford it, take heart. There are no guarantees, and they offer testimonials saying that the retreat has "helped many to manage this condition (FMS)" and some have "eliminated their symptoms completely."

were sick, but when they were well. Eastern doctors focus on achieving optimum health so the body can heal itself. Each patient has a different prognosis and different plan for recovery.

I begin to see how some of the alternative treatments that doctors dismiss (vitamins, colon cleanings, chiropractic, special diets, and so forth) could benefit some patients some times, not as placebos, but because they treat deficiencies or underlying conditions that Western medicine overlooks.

This makes perfect sense when you look at patient testimonies from those who live with incurable and largely untreatable diseases. Some of these nontraditional remedies help, not because they cure the disease, but because the sufferer has an underlying deficiency or medical problem that needs to be treated before the body can heal itself.

For example, some miracle cures consisting of massive doses of vitamins and minerals (often calcium, magnesium, and zinc) are effective with some patients. They didn't work for me, but they did for my younger sister, who suffers from asthma and chronic bronchitis. She has vastly improved with vitamin therapy and carries B and C vitamins in her purse, eating vitamins like candy. While she isn't cured, she feels much improved. But she's never been been much on nutrition. In general, the only vegetables she eats are onions and ketchup. It doesn't take a brain surgeon or even a GP to figure out that vitamins will improve the overall health of someone with vitamin deficiencies. In cases that aren't too severe, perhaps they may even lead to a cure. Because this sometimes happens, the bookshelves overflow with books exclaiming the virtues of vitamin therapy, and magazines and Web sites will cure you if you send them fistfuls of dollars for their specially balanced vitamin therapy. Of course, a balanced diet is cheaper, but who wants to be cured by eating carrots? And how could anyone make a fortune on it?

> **Tuning In**
>
> Music has been found to be a great pain reliever. According to a publication that reports on recent health care research, *The Cochrane Library*, 14 studies of 489 post-op patients found that music was second to medication in reducing pain. I keep an iPod next to my bed and play only happy or peaceful songs.

Similarly, chiropractors are often credited with miracle cures. If pain stems from a pinched nerve and the chiropractor removes the pressure, it's a miracle cure. Or if you're having a muscle spasm and a chiropractor can relieve it with a twist of the spine, then you may become a true chiropractic believer. But if you have something else, say, degenerative arthritis in the spine, you may decide that chiropractors are truly the quacks many doctors say they are.

Because these cures don't work for everyone, Western doctors don't recognize them as effective therapies. But everyone with a chronic illness should give the body all the help it needs in the form of vitamins, massage, chiropractic, rest, exercise, herbs, prayer, meditation, or whatever seems to help because a healthy body can fight back harder.

I believe fibromyalgia patients should read as many self-help books as they can with care and try to maintain optimum good health, but not every fibromyalgia patient will be cured or even vastly improved by vitamins, massage, acupuncture, or meditation. However, you might try massive doses of vitamin B, C, or E to see if they work. If you really need these vitamins, your body will let you know.

I read the books. I tried the therapies. I rearranged my schedule, exercised, rested, prayed, and swallowed calcium/magnesium tablets three times a day, and I did make some progress. Acupuncture was the best therapy, and it only alleviated the symptoms. And there is always the possibility that these therapies kept me from getting worse. It's hard to say. But I was disappointed, and these books ultimately led me to the same conclusion as some of my doctors. I must be doing something wrong. After all, if fibromyalgia can be controlled, as the doctors and some of the books insist, why couldn't I control my own?

More Eastern Alternatives

Yoga

Tai Chi

Meditation

Chi Chung (exercises to restore energy flow)

Fasting

Internal (colonic) cleansing

Unfortunately, acupuncture wasn't covered under our insurance, and it was expensive, $60 a treatment. In the beginning, I went three times a week. During the next three years, I went an average of once a week. Even though it put a dent on our savings account, I was lucky. Many fibromyalgia patients can't afford acupuncture.[3]

---

3   More and more insurance companies, recognizing the benefits, are beginning to cover it. If you have insurance and want to try acupuncture,

In the meantime, I rested and rested. I sipped odd and terrible-tasting herbal teas. Then one day in the spring, my acupuncturist told me to start exercising again. My pain level was down, but, to him, that wasn't the point. He knew it was time to start moving around because my pulse was getting stronger. Ah, the mysteries of Chinese medicine!

Don't be deterred if your doctor doesn't recommend acupuncture or chiropractic. Most alternative treatments are something else your doctor doesn't know about. And even if all you are getting is a placebo effect, so what? When my son played football, his coach wore the same T-shirt to every game. They won every game that season. Even if your confidence is restored by something that is likely nothing more than coincidence, what are you losing? Remember, you are for anything that makes you feel better, unless, of course, it is costing you an arm and a leg. So, if you believe that wearing a blue shirt will make you feel better, wear it. Please yourself. That's one thing that's sure to make you feel better.

I recommend calling your insurance company and making your case for acupuncture to them. I have had surprisingly good luck when I have called mine to discuss alternative treatments.

My vision is that every one of the nation's leading TV programs, radio broadcasts, magazines, and newspapers would report scientific evidence showing that followers of Jesus are three, four, or even five times healthier than those who don't believe in Jesus—that Christians have fewer incidents of cancer, heart disease, diabetes, and obesity. Wouldn't it be awesome if God's people were so full of good health, so vibrant, that others would notice us from ten or twenty feet away and wonder what our secret is?

Jordan Rubin, *The Great Physician's RX: 7 Weeks of Wellness Success Guide*

Chapter Seven

Praise the Lord and Pass the OxyContin

Once I was diagnosed with a mysterious and chronic illness, a strange thing happened. Medical practitioners of various faiths began to talk to me about religion. The first time it happened was in Chico, where I used to visit a chiropractor who believed in visitations from outer space. She was also a devout Christian. To keep her from proselytizing, I told her I was a Buddhist. My reasoning was that most evangelical Christians are trained to argue biblical scripture with Catholics, Protestants, and perhaps the Orthodox Church of Budapest as well, but they didn't know where to start if the potential convert doesn't accept the infallibility of the word of God, the Bible.

She liked me, so she was very sorry to hear I was a heathen, especially the part about me burning in hell because I didn't believe in Jesus. I told her not to worry about it. You could be a good Buddhist and still believe in Jesus as well.

"Maybe Jesus and Buddha and Confucius and Muhammad and Vishnu are all manifestations of the same divinity," I suggested as she straightened my back.

"Aha!" she said gleefully. "Then my god is stronger than your god because my god says he is the only true god while your god is made up of a lot of little gods."

There's nothing more demoralizing than a game of religious gotcha when you hurt so badly that you are having trouble staying focused. Too tired to argue, I generally left her office with spiritual tapes and fliers for upcoming revivals. Ordinarily, I would never have carried on a conversation with her, but she was oh so good when it came to straight-

69

ening out the kinks in my neck. Certainly, some god had given her a healing touch, although I always believed it was some heathen deity because, whatever god it was, it had a decidedly feminine touch.

She was only one of a number of health practitioners who preyed on my vulnerability. The chiropractor who replaced her, one with an office of Christian religious literature, had an unusual explanation for the cause of fibromyalgia.

"Well," he said, as his fingers probed the hard knots in my neck, "for the most part, only women get fibromyalgia. From my experience, it's women who resent their husbands. It's an unconscious thing really. They tend to be passive and submissive, but, in their hearts, they harbor a lot of anger."

I smiled. I wanted to laugh. No one in my entire life has ever described me as passive and submissive. Most of my life, there was no man in my life. I am aggressive and sharp-tongued to a fault.

"Hmmm," I said. "I don't think anyone I know would describe me as passive."

"You may not think you are," he said, "but you are. On the surface, you might be one person, but, deep down inside, you are someone else. That's where the pain comes from."

Undoubtedly, he wanted me to search deep inside and remove the mental roadblocks, like intelligence and independent thought, that prevented my wholehearted submission to my lord and husband. I didn't stay with the chiropractor for very long. Acupuncturist Maureen Lamerdin, a doctor of Oriental medicine, told me, as she rubbed my neck and shoulders after each treatment, that my neck was out.

"But I just went to the chiropractor," I protested over and over.

Finally, she said flat out one day, "You really need to find a new chiropractor."

I was happy to do so. The next chiropractor had religious literature all over his office as well, but he thought diet and exercise could improve fibromyalgia. He didn't talk to me about religion. Even better, he was buying a house with his girlfriend, and I was pretty sure he was living in sin. I'm not saying that was a good thing, but I did appreciate that he just tried to fix my neck and left my soul to my own discretion.

There are times when it is probably appropriate for doctors to discuss religion with their patients, but I would say that most of those times are when the patient initiates the conversation. Certainly, faith in a higher being and health are related. But when you are frightened and in pain, it's certainly presumptuous and uncomfortable when a medical professional tries to convert you to his or her religious persuasion.

Still, I was determined to try anything. In 2004, prayer and meditation were ranked as one of the most effective therapies at a Web site where patients rated their own treatments. This is no longer the case, and I can't begin to speculate on why this has changed. Perhaps it doesn't work as well as it did a few years ago. Maybe God is busy. Maybe he has gotten tired of fibromyalgia patients.

But many patients and doctors put their trust in prayer when they have no other answers. As I mentioned earlier, in at least one scientific study, patients who were prayed for fared much better in their recovery than a control group without a designated prayer group. Members of the prayer group did not know the patients; the patients did not know they were being prayed for. A second study did not duplicate these results. Who knows? Maybe the first group of spiritual contributors had better prayers. Maybe someone other than the recruited praying volunteers was praying for some of the patients without the scientist's knowledge or permission. One could, if one were a zealot, make the case that the outcome depended on which God the groups were praying to or whether God favored one group so he answered their prayers and simply ignored the others.

Some doctors believe only in lab results and diseases that make sense to them, leading them to conclude that, if they can't explain what is causing your pain, it must be all in your head. At the other extreme are doctors who believe God can cure cancer, alter your heart rhythms, and raise the (nearly) dead. Some doctors who can't cure you will have no qualms about imposing their spiritual beliefs on you. It's as if, when their white coats fail them, they don the dark, heavy robes of the priest and attempt to make the sign of the cross over your head.

I suppose every fibromyalgia patient has had at least one doctor who asked them about their religious beliefs and advised them to just put themselves in God's hands. I've had several, including the one whose only reading material in his office was the Bible.

I would have been happy to try religion, except I have always been kind of a skeptic and rarely a churchgoer. Getting a religion would be tough, especially if God can really read your mind when you are praying and knows you are wondering if he is out there and, if so, why he should cure you rather than use his energy to stop children from starving in Africa.

But even skeptics and nonbelievers know there is a spiritual element to suffering. In many religions, pain is a sacred ritual. "Whom the Lord loveth, He chasteneth." Remember how much God loved Job? In Christianity, the most dominant image is Jesus on the cross. We are supposed to suffer. In our literature, music, and stories handed down from one generation to another, heroes thrived because they suffered. They slew Beowulf's mother in a dreadful battle. They lost limbs in *Star Wars*. They were subjected to indignities and broken hearts in novels like *Pride and Prejudice*. And the pain and suffering somehow made them better, stronger, and purer in heart. So to what extent are we going against God's plan for us by relieving suffering with OxyContin and antidepressants?

In *The Truth about Chronic Pain*, Arthur Rosenfeld interviews June Dahl, PhD, professor of pharmacology and one of the architects of the Wisconsin Cancer Pain Initiative, about the correlation between the American bias against the use of pain medicine and the Puritan tradition. She says:

> If you look back on the history of our attitudes about pain and pain medicines in this country, you will find a lot of confusion. Surgeons used to think that pain was essential to healing.
>
> Most hospice workers will tell you that aggressive pain management probably prolongs life. Sometimes when family members call me because their loved ones won't take their medicine because they are afraid of being addicted to it, I'll say to the family member, "Look, pain is bad for you. There is evidence that your loved one will live longer if they take their medication." Somehow there is this perception that pain is a good thing, that it builds character. I don't see that pain has any redeeming virtues whatsoever. It destroys character.

But, having said this, I have to add that a few years ago, as Kevin and I hiked along one of Reno's snowy hills, reflecting on how our lives had changed with my illness, I asked if I had become a better person since I had been sick. He said yes. He said I have more humility and more sensitivity to others in pain. I argued that, when I was well, I had been more effective. As an editor, I was an advocate for the poor. There is an adage that the purpose of journalism is to comfort the afflicted and afflict the comfortable. I felt I had done both.

But Kevin disagreed. He said I may have been more powerful, but that power had also made me arrogant and less inclined to see the suffering in others and to respond to it. Even if I now had less obvious impact on the world in general, it didn't outweigh the fact that I had better intentions, less ambition, and more empathy. I don't like to think he is right. I hate every minute of my illness. Has it made me more spiritual?

Yes, I suppose it has. I certainly understand what it is like to live with chronic pain, and I am amazed to think that an estimated 50 million Americans live in chronic pain, according to the Academy of Pain Management. I once thought that chronic pain was mostly the domain of the elderly. Now I am much more aware that the man standing in line in front of me at the pharmacy counter walks with a slight limp, favoring one leg over another. I notice when a middle-aged woman shuffles slightly as she walks her dog down the street. When I see children in wheelchairs, I make a deliberate effort to catch their eye and smile because I know that people usually turn their heads, pretending they are invisible.

When I am driving and someone cuts in front of me, my anger sometimes dissipates when I think that he or she, like me, may be in excruciating pain every time he or she is at the wheel of his or her car. He or she may be hurrying simply to get to his or her destination as quickly as possible.

In the end, I did find some solace in religion in an unexpected way. I wanted to try meditation, so I went to those who were most famous for it, the Buddhists. I was relieved at my first meditation class that I did not have to be saved, recite a creed, or even speak to Buddha at all. All I had to do was sit cross-legged and try to concentrate on my breathing and listen to them explain a little bit about Buddhism. I learned the first noble truth is that all humans suffer and all of us long to avoid it. That sounded about right to me. Wasn't that what I was there for? To alleviate my pain?

I found the practice of quieting the mind helpful. It didn't always decrease my pain, but it made me less distressed by it. The teacher's constant focus on suffering as a universal quality of all mankind helped me to be less bitter and recognize that many others suffered more than I did. In fact, I really had nothing to be sorry for. I was fifty-four years old. I was a college graduate and the mother of three stunning, successful children who were healthy and happy. I had already outlived the average life span of most human beings, given that, in Afghanistan, the normal life span today is forty-seven. Less than one thousand years ago, the average European never lived to see his or her grandkids. I had flown in airplanes, watched on television while men walked on the moon, and traveled all over the United States. I had watched the sunset over the Pacific Ocean and the Gulf of Mexico. I had danced all night and feasted all day. I had been to Paris. I had reached career goals I had set for myself as a teenager. I had taught college classes. I had written for national magazines. I had published poetry.

More Ideas

Massage

Acupressure

Water aerobics

Hot tubs

Rebounding (working on a small trampoline)

Rolfing (a type of massage)

Biofeedback

Allergy testing

Two scoops of your favorite ice cream!

When a fifty-four-year-old woman develops an incurable pain syndrome, it is, as a friend phrased it, "more than a bit of bad luck." But it is not a tragedy. When a seven-year-old starves to death or a ten-year-old dies of leukemia, that's a tragedy. If I knew I was going to die tomorrow, I would have to admit that I had already lived a rich, full life.

But would I trade my spiritual growth if I could suddenly get well tomorrow? You bet I would. I know it sounds terrible, but it's true. This isn't suffering that I willingly took on as part of a self-improvement campaign.

If I got well tomorrow, would I forget within a few years, weeks, or even days what is it to be in chronic pain? Would I quickly turn away from others who were suffering because I would not want to be reminded of my own illness?

I sincerely hope not, but it's hard to say. In the end, linking pain to growth opens the door to some pretty crazy notions. If we know that pain is good for personal growth, shouldn't we inflict it on everyone? And who is to say that my personal growth was simply a result of my growing older and becoming more mature? Pain didn't immediately transform me into a better human being. It sometimes turned me into a cranky bitch. In fact, it's likely that, for every serene, loving person in pain, three or four miserable wretches try to make others suffer as they do.

My meditation helped with my sour moods and temper tantrums, but not enough. I have always had a bad temper, but now I had a terrible one. Even though I was taking antidepressants, I would be strong and resilient one minute and furious and frustrated the next. On bad days, I was often pretty silent until Kevin asked me to run to the store or bring him a Diet Coke from the kitchen. Then I would blow up. How dare he ask me to wait on him when I was in such incredible pain!

"How do I know when you are feeling really bad if you don't tell me?" he asked.

He had a point. I tried harder to communicate with him. He also began to pay more attention to my silences. If I was quiet or cross, he would ask, "Is this a bad pain day?"

That's what we called them. Every day was labeled: bad pain day, good day, or okay day. Good days didn't mean there was no pain, only that I could function at a level closer to normal. We later refined the system and used a one-to-ten pain meter, with ten being natural childbirth or passing a kidney stone. As time went by, Kevin began to take the initiative, asking me the moment I woke up to give him some feedback on my pain level.

He also commented when I was in a good mood. His feedback was invaluable. I began to realize how closely my pain level determined my state of mind. Instead of finding that a good mood would keep down my pain, I found that a low pain level elevated my mood. Maybe this is what makes positive thinking so easy for some and so difficult for others. Frankly, those

You're Not Alone

It's estimated that 50 million Americans suffer from chronic pain.

with a positive attitude may not be in as much pain as they think they are. Pain is a subjective thing. Someone who rates their pain as very high but keeps a positive outlook may not be suffering as much as someone who rates their pain as high, but not very high. Who knows which one really has more pain? I'm sure most of us think our pain is less tolerable than someone else's. If you listen to women talk about childbirth, it's a rare woman who admits to an easy delivery.

Perhaps the conversation I dislike the most is when someone tries to argue that he or she suffers more than you do. This is even worse than those who believe that what you really have are a few aches and pains of old age creeping in, even if you're thirty. But as for those who have to prove that their pain is worse than yours, I can't really believe they have ever suffered very deeply because, once you have, you will never think of level of anguish as a contest you would like to win.

In fact, you know there are no winners when pain becomes disabling, and it is hard to feel anything but sympathy for those who have suffered as much you have. My sister, who is not a saint but lives with constant misery, says she doesn't want FMS to happen to her worst enemy. I am no angel either, but I have to say that, whenever I hear of anyone who has fibromyalgia, I am saddened, especially when children as young as four or five years old are diagnosed with it.

Ask about TENS Units

These small machines deliver an electric current that interrupts pain messages to the brain. Like acupuncture, they are highly effective for some, but not all, pain patients.

But there are still too many doctors out there who prefer patients with smiles and long-suffering attitudes to those screaming in agony and who believe the only difference between the two groups is not the pain level but the patient's disposition. It's easy for them to prescribe a good attitude, but you can't fill a prescription for happiness.

If patients could cure chronic pain with positive thinking, what a different world it would be. Psychologists can prove that pain is linked to states of mind, like depression, despair, nervousness, jitters, and a host of other mental conditions, but they can't explain why some depressed patients never experience any physical pain or why some patients in chronic pain still have positive outlooks.

If you have chronic pain or fibromyalgia, you have heard at least one pep talk, as if you could talk yourself out of the disease. You can't talk yourself out of a toothache, a broken kneecap, a migraine, or a hangover. You can't talk yourself out of fibromyalgia either. Don't put up with any doctor who tells you otherwise.

Don't let someone who hasn't been in your shoes try to make you feel responsible for your illness. Most of us already try too hard to think ourselves well. Remind yourself that you are doing the best you can.

Do try to think positive that there are better days ahead, but don't force yourself to carry out your daily responsibilities cheerfully while you are in terrible pain. Let others know when you don't feel well. You may sometimes want company; you may want to be alone other times.

It helps if you have a friend who has chronic pain that you can call when you want to vent and feel that someone else understands you. Calling a friend who is sympathetic and not judgmental is one of the best stress relievers I have found. But, as far as I'm concerned, you should hang up on anyone who tries to give you a lecture. You didn't ask for this. You have to cope with a difficult condition, and you can't just wish it away.

A Simple Meditation

Sit in a comfortable posture. Close your eyes. Breathing slowly and evenly, count each breath. When you get to ten, start over. Try to focus on your breathing. Feel the air as it moves through your nasal passages, through your trachea, and into your lungs. After several minutes, when you feel relaxed, imagine that soothing light rays are beaming down on you, clearing away all thought and anxiety. You may not feel them at first, and your mind will wander off. Just keep bringing your thoughts back to the rays. If you feel distracted by pain in a particular place, concentrate on the pain, and focus on the warm light that is healing it. If the pain moves somewhere else, follow it with your mind. Try to find the pain and soothe it instead of ignoring it.

Work is a necessity for people with fibromyalgia just as it is with almost everyone else.

Fibromyalgia: A Comprehensive Approach

Chapter Eight

Your Job Is Not Your Best Therapy

Over the years, doctors, chiropractors, physician assistants, other fibromyalgia patients, and even members of my own family have lectured me about the importance of keeping my job. I am told that work "keeps your mind off the pain." Unfortunately, depending on its severity, pain can keep your mind off work. But no one ever says that.

Then, of course, there is always a story or anecdote about a friend or co-worker who has fibromyalgia and continues to work full-time because he or she loves his or her job so much. "It's good therapy." The implication being that, if you don't work, you don't like your job and are just looking for an excuse to quit.

Truthfully, if you are struggling to keep a full-time job, you may be seriously hurting yourself. Rest is often rated first on the list by patients who evaluate their own treatments at online sites. For five years, I struggled with a series of jobs, searching for one that would accommodate my illness. I was obsessed with working. When I wasn't working, I juiced up carrots, celery, and kale for my morning pick-me-up, dragged myself up hills during my morning walk, and

---

Midnight Madness

Working at night or staying awake for any reason between the hours of 1:00 and 5:00 AM can have an extremely deleterious effect on your health. Most of us are programmed to rest and repair our bodies at this time. Consequently, our defenses are low. We don't think clearly and are easily disturbed and distressed. If you wake up and cannot get back to sleep after fifteen to thirty minutes, get out of bed, watch TV, read a book, surf the Web, listen to movies, and indulge in a snack. If you are depressed or anxious, remind yourself that you are not at your best and things will look better in the morning.

---

read self-help books for fibro patients in the bathtub, all with my eye on one thing, going back to work.

I didn't do this because of the feelings of guilt and inadequacy that medical experts, friends, and family imposed on me. I wanted to work. I wanted the prestige. I wanted the money. I wanted to keep writing and editing until I died. I wanted to die like George Bernard Shaw, who died from complications after he fell out of a tree he was trimming. He was ninety-four and in the middle of writing a new play and reorganizing the English language.

I didn't need a pep talk. Before I got sick, I was a walking pep talk. I desperately needed doctors to tell me to slow down, stop, sleep, and rest. I was later diagnosed with sleep apnea, and I was horrified to think of the damage I had done to my body and my weary brain as I kept forcing it into higher and higher levels of performance when the only thing that could have healed me was deep sleep. I hadn't had a good night's sleep in years, maybe in decades.

I often fantasize about suing my former doctors for malpractice. Not only did they miss the obvious signs of sleep apnea, they insisted the best therapies were exercise and work. This is probably part of our American culture. We can never slow down, and we suspect anyone who doesn't own a treadmill or belong to a gym is a closet Baskin-Robbins addict with a TV remote in hand six hours a day.

For people who are capable of exercise, there's no doubt about its benefits. But exercise and overwork create dangerous health conditions, especially if you are overweight or out of shape or have high blood pressure or sleep apnea.

Doctors, friends, and families also tend to underestimate the severity of the pain of fibromyalgia, perhaps because doctors sometimes label any unexplained aches or pains as fibromyalgia, so people who tell you they have fibromyalgia may have a bit of mild discomfort that comes and goes. Maybe some people do have very mild cases. I have heard others say they heard that fibromyalgia "really doesn't hurt that bad." And I know I have been treated by doctors who feel the same way.

For those of you without fibromyalgia who might be reading this, let me explain. It feels like rigor mortis setting in while you are still alive. Your muscles and joints are turning to brick, squeezing the nerve endings and prompting them to pulse frantically, as if it were possible that you could do something to help them. It sometimes feels as if the bones themselves hurt, as if they are too hard for the soft tissue around them and as if the bones were concrete rods strung through your body.

Other times, the muscles form bands of tiny knots. You can feel them if you run your fingers down your arm or leg, and these small bands sometimes form a giant muscle spasm. Others have described the pain as fire. For me, it has more the texture of hot coals, which sometimes cause my whole body to break out into a sweat. In some ways, it is worse than the pain because nothing, not an ice bag, cold water, or even cold shower, can counter the all-encompassing heat. Droplets bubble up like steamy dew on my forehead and between my breasts and run down my neck, even though I never sweated much before my illness. Ten years ago, I had to run for a mile before I broke a sweat. But, with fibromyalgia, I don't have to move off the couch. At the same time that my upper body radiates like an oven, my feet are as cold and stiff as glaciers. It's like all the blood and heat is in my head and trunk, leaving nothing to warm my feet and legs. I put ice packs on my neck and woolen socks on my feet. It's frightening to realize your body is unable to regulate itself. It can no longer decide whether it is too hot and too cold, and pain, nausea, and dizziness overwhelm me.

Even when my symptoms first appeared, mornings were generally the worst. If you have ever slept on a slab of concrete and woke up nearly unable to move, you may be able to get a glimmer of what I am talking about. Everything hurt as I moved. I felt like an old piece of farm equipment, rusted and rigid. I often rolled my head from side to side, encouraging the muscles to relax, and then lifted my legs, rolled my shoulders, bent my elbows, and brought my hands to my shoulders, as if I were lifting imaginary weights. My hands, made worse by a touch of osteoarthritis, were hot and swollen. I curled my fingers in and out, hoping to relieve the stiffness. The first few steps after I climbed out of bed were miserable and uneven. I made tea, took anti-depressants, and popped a couple Vicodin. If I was not too hot, I might immerse myself to the chin in hot water. If I was hot, I used an ice pack on my neck. Other times, I just walked around the room in circles, trying to get the blood to circulate.

Over the last few years, I have added too many words for pain to my vocabulary: searing, stinging, agonizing, piercing, throbbing, grinding, excruciating, nauseating, and gnawing. And these are just the adjectives.

Oddly, unlike other painful conditions like childbirth, where fellow sufferers often compete, trying to convince their listeners that their experience is the most harrowing, fibromyalgiacs take no comfort in knowing that their pain dwarves all others. As symptoms occur, they ask each other, "Did you ever have the feeling where—" There's solace in knowing that someone else shares these strange and nearly indescribable sensations, yet we don't want to outdo each other. We secretly hope we are doing better than anyone else is.

Of course, if you can work, I know you don't have to be told to keep your job. It's a pretty rare individual who would prefer staying home drawing a pittance in disability, if, of course, you manage to collect disability. Again, I think this is a cultural myth that, given a choice, we all want to stay home and watch Oprah.

During the two years I taught at a community college, I did not improve. In fact, being in a classroom became increasingly uncomfortable, and I would have to rest after teaching just one hour. If there was an incident in class, including a smart-aleck student, lost notes, or an after-class discussion over a grade, my body would tense up, and the pain spiked.

Finally, against the advice of my doctors, I decided to take a break for a year to try to heal myself. The only physician who didn't disagree with me was the family physician who had treated me during the twelve years I lived in Chico. I went to visit him when I was in town and told him I was planning to take some time off. Even though I knew I needed the rest, I guess I was still a bit disappointed when he agreed with me.

"Work is overrated, Linda," he said. In the end, of course, he was right.

I filed for disability, crying all the way through the interview process. It was clearly not the way I wanted to end my career. This was something that wasn't supposed to happen to me. I took care of myself, exercised, and ate the right foods. I had spent my life getting an education and building a career. I felt helpless and dependent.

"She doesn't look disabled to me."

How many times had I heard someone say that? Maybe I had even said it myself. Maybe you have, too. You're driving around the parking lot in the rain, looking for a place to park, and you see a middle-aged woman pull her SUV into a handicapped spot and hop out. Pretty soon, that woman would be me. I didn't look disabled. I didn't limp or wince whenever I took a step. I didn't use a cane or a walker. But there were days when a reduction of ten steps was a lifesaver.

I stayed at home for nearly a year. And I did improve. From the beginning, every acupuncturist I had consulted had encouraged me to rest, and I finally took their advice. Unlike American medical doctors who find treating fibromyalgia frustrating and unpleasant, Maureen, my favorite acupuncturist, listened with interest. When she insisted that I forget about exercising and rest as much as possible, I thought long and hard about it. Intuitively, I felt it was what my body needed to do at that time.

A Japanese masseuse had once told me, "Listen to your body." Because the medical advice given to me by GPs so far was at best confusing and at worst seemed to increase my pain and distress, I decided to just do whatever my body seemed to want to do. There was no more forcing or working through exhaustion. Maureen's advice made sense.

She also believed I could recover. She gave me something to hope for. As the months went by and I improved, I began to feel better, and I came to trust her and value her advice. When she told me to rest, I rested. I felt she was a true healer, not a shaman or psychic. She was just someone who was good at evaluating my condition as the symptoms waxed and waned. She could not cure my fibromyalgia, but she helped me to strengthen my body and mind, diminish the pain temporarily, and learn to deal with it when it happened. Thankfully, many alternatives can decrease pain and help you get back into a regular exercise regime, which will help you improve even more. With FMS, you are either on a downward spiral or an upward staircase, and alternative medicine and treatments have turned me back in the right direction in many cases. In a few months after I started seeing Maureen, I signed up for tap dancing lessons, taking my place in the front row with about a dozen middle-aged women who still remembered how it felt to be little girls. It sometimes did make me a little sore afterwards, but the lift it gave my spirits made it worthwhile.

Many wise and experienced doctors who are highly trained in fibromyalgia agree with my acupuncturist. Dr. Alina Garcia, a fibromyalgia specialist in Las Vegas, told me, "Exercise is a two-edged sword … When you exercise you make more mitochondria, which can be a good thing, or it can exhaust your adrenals."

She continues to say that only by thorough and exhaustive tests, evaluations, and monitoring can effective treatments be found. Fibromyalgia treatments do not come in one-size-fits-all.

◆   ◆   ◆

Years after my diagnosis, Kevin took a job in Reno, and I got an unsolicited call from the senior editor at the *Reno Gazette-Journal*, asking if I were interested in applying for a part-time job editing a weekly section. I decided to try it. I had a two-day audition for the job, where I edited and pulled together a few pages, but, after the first few hours on the first day, I knew I couldn't come back. I could not sit at a desk for hours on end.

"Just call him and tell him the truth," Kevin said that night as I eased myself into a tub of hot water.

Telling the truth seems like a simple thing to do. Every time I told someone I couldn't work, I felt like I was resigning from my career forever. I was also afraid the word would get out. Because of what we do, newspapers have an amazing network. When I was well enough to work full-time, a prospective employer would hear gossip. I had this weird condition that had transformed me from an outstanding editor to a worker's comp claim just waiting to happen.

The truth is, back in my old days as editor, I would not have hired someone with fibromyalgia. Sounds pretty awful, doesn't it? I once hired a superb entry-level journalist who called in sick two months after she was hired to tell me she had chronic fatigue syndrome. I was furious that she hadn't told me before she came on board. Sure, maybe you shouldn't discriminate, but who wants to train someone for six months only to have him or her resign? Worse, who wants to hire someone who can only produce about 50 percent of what he or she should, especially when newspapers are notoriously short-staffed and most employees work about 150 percent more than they should have to?

Now I was faced with the problem from a different angle, and I decided I needed to tell the truth about why I was declining the job. My prospective boss was extremely understanding. He said he was sorry to hear that, but he still wanted to hire me as a freelance writer.

But even that proved pretty exhausting. I generally didn't get my assignments until Monday, and they were due on Wednesday morning.

Some days were good; other days were miserable. I was on the phone and at the computer all day. It took the rest of the week to recover.

One day, Kevin, who was working as a copy editor, suggested he read my copy before I turned it in.

"Don't you have enough to read?" I asked him.

With a sad, embarrassed frown, he said he worried about my brain fog. Journalists aren't expected to make stupid mistakes, at least not many. And one stupid mistake can lead to a lawsuit. I was hurt, but I had to admit he was right. Mental confusion and the urgency of deadlines were a bit more than I could handle.

"Okay," I told myself, "so maybe I can't be a journalist anymore."

Of course, there was always teaching. But that was getting more difficult as well. From the first, I had difficulties in staying organized. A few times, I was busy talking to Kevin in the afternoon and nearly forgot to go to class.

Talk about forgetful! How can you forget to go to work? I asked Kevin to remind me when I needed to start getting ready, and God help him if he forgot. Once again, he was to blame for my problems.

This kind of carelessness was totally unlike me. I was usually overly prompt and spent the last hour before class going over notes and so forth. Now I was running out of the house, praying that I had grabbed the right books and my notes were somewhere in one of the files I picked up. As my mind became less capable of organizing, I tried to become more outwardly organized. I used to throw papers around, stack things on my desk, leave books in my car, but no more. I color-coded my files, stapled lecture notes to the inside of folders, and wrote notes in the index of books. As it was, I occasionally lost my lecture notes right in the middle of the lecture. You can only shuffle papers on your desk so many times in front of your students without looking like you've lost your mind as well, so I would wing it, only to find later that I had tucked my notes into a file with students' papers I planned to return.

I spent an inordinate amount of time going through student papers, making sure I hadn't lost or misfiled them, always sure I would lose some. In the past, when a student insisted, as they sometimes do, that he or she had turned in a paper I hadn't seen, I knew he or she was lying. Now I wasn't so sure.

I also had trouble checking my mail. The part-time faculty mailboxes were on the other side of campus. On particularly painful days, I didn't make the hike. My students generally e-mailed late assignments, but I was embarrassingly late in responding to correspondence from the English department. But with note cards and Post-It notes everywhere, I managed to get through the semester.

The Best Acupuncture

Doctors can claim to be acupuncturists if they take a weekend class in acupuncture. It's best to ask how much training your acupuncturist has had. Those trained in Asia have generally spent years perfecting their craft, and some Americans who are not doctors have years of training. Acupuncture is more like an art than a medical procedure. Find the best you can in your area.

Terrified, knowing I was faltering and couldn't really do the job, I turned on Kevin. He finished work around 12:30 and came home at 1:00 AM. Then he spent an hour or two unwinding before he went to bed. He often didn't get to bed until about 3:00. If he accidentally awakened me on a night when I had managed to sleep past midnight, I became hysterical, screaming, yelling, and stomping around the house. Mean? You bet. In those dark hours, I was exhausted and frantic. I feared that one more lost night's sleep would cost me my job. Once again, Kevin and I began to sleep in separate beds.

I can't imagine I was helping anyone by forcing myself through each excruciating day at work. Sure, I felt more important than when I was sitting at home, but I paid a high price for those fleeting feelings of self-esteem.

We had a six-week break over Christmas. The snow that had lingered for almost two months had disappeared, and I began to take long walks with Kevin and our dogs. I doubled up on acupuncture and spent my days resting.

Acupuncture often makes me pleasantly drowsy. I sometimes fall asleep. My limbs often tingle. But, one day, on one of my more painful days, during the session, the tingling began to turn into a delicious sensation, as if my body had turned into a running brook. I felt no pain at all, just a soft, flowing sensation that was almost electric, from my tingling scalp to my toes. After a minute or two of pure enjoyment, I wondered what was going on. In fact, I wondered if I were dead. If I were, I reasoned I didn't mind because it felt so good. I had absolutely no pain.

But just as I was really relaxing and enjoying it, I became aware once again of the pain in my hips, the muscle spasm in my back, my stiff neck, and sore legs. Yep, I was alive all right, and the flowing sensation subsided.

Maureen came in a few minutes later. "How are you doing?"

"Okay," I said, "but this is kind of trippy."

She listened, nodding happily as I explained what I had felt.

"That's a wonderful sign," she said. "You are going to get well."

When school started in January, I was on the mend. Fortunately, my schedule that semester wasn't as demanding.

One day, I noticed it was hardly an effort to tramp across campus to get my mail. I began to walk up the stairs to my classroom instead of waiting for the elevator. I was much more coherent in the classroom. It was clear I was in remission. I began to have hope again. It made sense to me that, if I could feel well for a day or even a few hours, my body had the potential to restore itself to set things right, even if temporarily. If I felt good for a day, why couldn't I feel well for a week, a month, a year, or forever?

The next semester passed uneventfully. For those four months, I was at a place where my part-time job was not debilitating or exhausting. I finished the classes. Kevin and I went to Europe on vacation, and I came back ready for a bigger challenge, especially after we climbed the steps up the Eiffel Tower. Climbing the tower, I was a slow starter, and I sometimes had to rest, so we stopped to let others pass. But when we arrived at the first tier, the view was magnificent. Was it worth attempting the second? In a half hour or so, I was there, looking out over the city. Kevin wanted to attempt the third, but the long line discouraged him. For me, the second tier was a complete victory. I felt as if I had conquered the city, perhaps even Europe itself. Most of all, at that moment, I realized my life didn't have to be over, even if it meant living with constant pain. There would still be days when I was on top of the world or, at least, on top of Paris.

I was done teaching part-time. I felt I was ready to get back into journalism. Looking back, I can see I had read too many positive-thinking self-help books on fibromyalgia and consulted too many doctors who extolled the benefits of work as therapy. Even Maureen thought returning to work as a journalist was worth a try. There was no one to stop me from hurting myself.

One way to go into business for yourself is to think of all the things you'd pay someone to do for you, then pick one or two and offer to do them for other people ... No matter how much you think you have lost, there are plenty of things you can do. Try. Take chances. You'll surprise yourself, and enrich your life and the lives of others as well.

Fibromyalgia: A Comprehensive Approach

Chapter Nine

The Fibro Fantasy: I'm As Well As I Want To Be

About this time, my former boss from the *Paradise Post*, Lowell Blankfort, approached me with the idea of starting our own publication. I was full of bluster and exaggerated vigor. I had convinced myself that riding a bicycle for forty-five minutes was the equivalent of full-time work.

Blankfort is a sensible businessman who didn't understand the depths of my illness, but my husband did, and he didn't like it one bit.

"What if you get sick again?" he asked repeatedly.

I had tried five jobs in the last three years. Why would I think this would work? I quoted from the fibromyalgia bibles about how much easier it is to have your own business when you have fibromyalgia because you can control your work hours, cut back on bad days, and work harder on good ones. You can hire someone to fill in on bad days.

Of course, I knew this was pure bunk. Running your own business, with perhaps a few exceptions, is more stressful, more exhausting, and more demanding than working for someone else. There are things you can't delegate. There are times when you have to show up. There are money worries, deadline worries, and production worries. You can't call in sick on bad days if you have to soothe an irate customer. You don't have a boss to answer to, but you have clients who can be even more unreasonable.

I suspect that the only reason most fibromyalgia guides suggest self-employment is because it works for those who provide certain types

> **Warning!**
>
> Nothing can be more dangerous to your health than a doctor who assures you that you are able to work when you can hardly get out of the bed in the morning.

of services, like bookkeepers or freelance writers like me. But does it work for doctors in emergencies, accountants at tax time, or babysitters when a mom has to work late? Will the IRS give you a break because your bookkeeping isn't up-to-date? Will it work for housecleaners who can't find an address or can't move the couch to vacuum underneath?

But I wanted to do this so badly that I was ready to mortgage our house. It was just a small mortgage. I assured my husband that it couldn't fail. But he wouldn't budge.

"Okay, okay, maybe not mortgage the house," I relented.

Maybe we could start the paper on a shoestring, make a minimal investment, and work some long hours. It was the first true remission I had, and I felt like I was about 80 percent better. I didn't know that remissions could last for months or years. I thought they lasted forever. I wanted to write my own book on coping with fibromyalgia. I felt like the acupuncture, carrot juice, positive thinking, and all those wonderful books had not only helped me improve, I felt I was on my way to a permanent cure. I was going to be one of those rare ones.

The one condition that did not improve was insomnia, for which I took Valium, and I sometimes napped in the afternoon. But the pain that had once dominated my life pain was now a background irritant, like a mild toothache. I could live with that. Oh boy, could I live with that.

And I was still getting better. Nearly every day, I rode my bike or hiked up and down a hill near our house for an hour. Sure, it always hurt, especially uphill, but after a year or two of chronic pain, you can gauge the intensity of the pain by how distracting it is. When the pain level drops, you are almost oblivious to it. If someone asks you if it hurts, you'd say, "Yeah, sure."

But it's almost like you have to think about it for a minute. It's buried there somewhere, like an old T-shirt under a pile of clothes in a dresser drawer. During a flare-up, on the other hand, it's impossible to think of anything else. If someone asks you what you have been doing all day, your first thought is that you have been hurting. You may not even remember anything else, like what you had for lunch, whom you talked to, or what you said.

And I still had bad nights, nights where I woke up with horrible, wracking pain, not knowing if I would sleep the rest of the night. It was often like being chased through a nightmare by the furies of hell.

Sometimes, even the Valium didn't work, and I would sit up in bed all night, reading.

Sitting up in bed reading all night sounds more peaceful and predictable than it was. When I woke up, it was as if something had jarred me awake, something dangerous and threatening. These symptoms had started when I was a child. I can remember waking up at 2:00 or 3:00 AM in the morning and not being able to get back to sleep. For this reason, my parents considered me a nervous child, with nightmares and frequent awakenings as a symptom of overstimulation.

I shared a bed with my younger sister, and I can remember lying next to her, listening to her even breathing. Some nights, I cried in frustration. Other times, I was terrified. On at least one occasion, I woke up my sister to tell her I was dying. I was certain I was. She would stumble out of bed to wake up my mother, who, more often than not, was clearly annoyed by my midnight bids for attention.

As an adult, there were a few times when I couldn't sleep for days at a time. The first time it happened, I was under a lot of stress. A guy I was dating had just dumped me. Lying awake and pining for an unrequited love, that's happened to lots of us if you believe the love songs on the radio. But, other times, I laid awake all night long for no reason I could explain. It happened again the next year, almost exactly one year later. Shortly before I started working in journalism, I went for three days without sleeping and began to hallucinate. I was walking around the house at midnight, in a state of panic, sure that Jack the Ripper was lurking outside my bedroom window.

As I walked through the living room, I noticed a pile of newspapers in the middle of the floor. As I stooped to pick them up, the papers began to move. I reached for them again, and they moved across the room. As I straightened up on my shaking knees, I realized I was trying to tidy up my dog. Very quietly and solemnly, I sat down in my favorite chair and waited for dawn to come. I knew I was hallucinating, and I was afraid to get up for fear of hurting myself. I don't remember if I dozed at all. It was one of the many longest nights of my life.

When dawn came, a friend drove me to the emergency room. The doctor gave me six sleeping pills and told me to take one every two hours until I fell asleep. At 4:00 PM, the third pill knocked me out. I asked all my doctors, my family doctor, gynecologist, and allergy specialist what could have caused this, and no one had an answer for me. They said it was just some odd quirk or stress.

But I had insomnia when I was happy and when I was depressed. I've had it when I was somewhere between happiness and depression. It was like menstruation. It came and went.

Migraines followed pretty much the same pattern, none. Sure, stress affects our body rhythms. Who doesn't feel blissful and alive in a sailboat on the Pacific on a sunny day with a gentle breeze keeping you cool? Someone who gets seasick, that's who. But does stress cause seasickness? Would it cause you to get sunburned? No. Doctors see a pattern there, and they can explain it. Anything else they can't explain is driven by stress. I sometimes think it's the stress of their own lives that makes them see stress everywhere, something like Freud did with sex.

The hours between 1:00 and 5:00 AM are not a happy time, unless you are young and intoxicated with wine or love. For me, it was the loneliest time in the world, as well as the most frightening, although the fear may have been driven by the not-quite-conscious but very certain notion that something was terribly wrong.

So the insomnia continued. As odd as this may seem, it reinforced my idea that being in business for myself might be the best solution. I would often creep out of bed at 2:00 AM and begin researching vendors, designing pages, or writing lists of story ideas. It assuaged my anxiety and gave me something to do until I began to get sleepy as the sun came up. Then I would nap until about 9:00 AM. Because most

---

**To Work Or Not To Work …
That Is The Question.**

Deciding whether to keep your job depends on many other factors besides how much pain you can endure and still be functional. You will also have to consider:

Do you have sufficient control of your bladder and bowels?

Can you live with yourself if your co-workers resent you when you are not pulling your weight?

Will your boss support you, or will he or she secretly feel you avoid doing unpleasant tasks because of your disability?

Are you making enough money to pay for extra massages and/or acupuncture you may need?

Will your disability affect your job performance reviews?

Will the stress of your job deplete your energy to the point that you will no longer have energy for your family or other activities?

businesses who would buy ads in my paper opened at 10:00, I reasoned I'd be starting my workday as they were unlocking their doors and flipping over their Open signs.

I could also control my schedule a bit more. Although I knew it meant long hours and lots of headaches, I could, in a real pinch, reschedule an appointment or work long hours on good days and shorten my days when I had to.

Maureen, my acupuncturist, took more than my physical pulse when I went for treatment. She charted my progress and would sometimes read the notes from my previous visits so I could see how far I had come. She felt that, with a reasonable schedule, I was ready for a bigger challenge.

On my daily walks, I thought about business almost all the time, thinking of pitches to use for new customers, how to set up my accounting, and what to charge for advertising. Through the long nights, I read books on sales and starting small businesses and newspaper design and home improvement. During the day, I discussed plans with Lowell.

Kevin never got on board. "What if you get sick again?" he repeated like a mantra.

Sure, I admitted that could be a disaster, but it didn't matter. It wasn't going to happen. Hadn't I made consistent progress over the last two years? I was hiking, biking, and working out with Richard Simmons tapes. I was an oldie but goodie, sweating with the over-fifty crowd.

Kevin's lack of confidence didn't deter me. I was used to forging ahead without the support of my closest friends and family members. Did I listen when I first told my mother that I wanted to be a writer, and she suggested I set my sights on something much more practical, like learning to cut hair? Did I listen when she told me I couldn't go to college, that I should be happy to have a husband with a blue-collar job who paid the bills? My whole family surely thought I was crazy when, at thirty-three, I quit the first decent job I'd ever had, working as a field representative for a printing company, to go to graduate school and get a master's degree in English literature.

About the only person I listened to at this point was Maureen. She thought I could work if I took care of myself. In my morning walks surrounded by desert wildflowers, I promised myself that I would still manage to put myself first, to attend to my health above everything.

Seeing that he wasn't getting anywhere, Kevin suggested I at least check out other options before jumping into business for myself. Why not try a part-time job in journalism for a few months or even a year or two to see if my progress was permanent? Why did I have to jump into this so quickly?

As a concession to him, I e-mailed the editor at the *Reno Gazette-Journal* who had interviewed me the previous year and told him I didn't intend to return to teaching. I felt I was well enough to return to journalism. Did they have any part-time or freelance openings?

He replied immediately, suggesting I apply for the job opening as features editor. Still determined to go it alone and convinced my own business would be more manageable than a real job, I put him off.

Scheduling

Most FMS patients are worse in the morning and at night. If this is true for you, try to schedule your work or errands for the middle of the day. Even doctors' appointments are best at times when you are alert and at your best.

Kevin was not the only skeptic at this point. There were days when I felt pretty bad, days when I could hardly sit at the computer, days when I had to skip aerobics, and times when I spaced things out. But, as I began to worry, Kevin vacillated, sometimes supportive of what Lowell and I were doing and, at other times, warning me that I could just be in a temporary remission.

"What's going to happen if you get sick again?" he asked. "You don't have anyone to back you up. It's a lot of work and lot of pressure."

More and more, my confidence wavered. Once I went to meet with a potential advertiser who installed ponds. I hadn't slept at all the previous night, despite several milligrams of Valium. I had woken up feeling worse than if I had drank a bottle of vodka and twice as tired. My head ached. I hurt all over. I couldn't think straight, and my eyes were red and swollen, as if I had been crying. Determined not to let a bad night ruin a productive day, I went anyway. The owner was late, which meant I stood in the hot Reno sun for nearly an hour, sweating and in serious pain. When he finally showed up, he insisted on marching me all over the store. Because I viewed him as an expectant advertiser, I feigned an interest in the fifty different kinds of fish that fill backyard ponds. When I asked about pictures, he sent me to his stepson, who took another hour or so to download photos onto a CD.

By the end of the interview, my knees were shaking. I came home and went to bed. Luckily, Kevin was about to leave for work, so he didn't realize how sick I was.

But he was hard to fool. Most days, he could tell how I was feeling. By now, he was aware of the slightest change in facial color, vocal tone, and expression. So there was no putting on a happy face for my husband. The face I wore was what I was feeling. Even though he had been delighted with my progress, he knew how often I was faking it.

And he knew when I slept or didn't sleep. He worked nights and came home in the middle of the night. He'd sometimes find me propped up on pillows, reading *Ivanhoe* for the twenty-third time. He could always tell when I was on the ropes. He knew that, even in remission, I still had serious symptoms.

Was I worried? Sure, but I was more worried about becoming an invalid and a burden on him than on the stress I would put on my body. I was determined to make this work, and I would. End of story.

In the long run, Kevin rescued me from the positive thinking I had adopted after overdosing on feel-good fibromyalgia folklore, and his stubbornness saved me from myself. I resented him at times because I thought he was trying to hold me back. Only later did I decide that he was the one person who was trying to protect me.

Of course, he didn't know that I had my own doubts. I was already working out contingency plans in case I was bedridden. Could I hire someone to do the writing on the cheap? Could I communicate with clients via phone calls, fax, and e-mails if I were too sick to go in person? Could I get a part-time secretary/bookkeeper?

I think a lot of my ability to compete. I work hard, and I am not easily deterred if I am in stubborn pursuit of something I want. But I also knew that, even with all the street smarts and willpower in the world, someone who is about to open a business had better have both feet on the ground, not as I had at that minute. Both feet were propped up on the rail of the backyard swing while I lay on my back.

I told him I would think about it. And I did. For a week or so, I trudged up and down the steep hill just blocks from my house. How can you be objective about your own health? And how can you predict the course of a disease that baffles doctors so much so that many doctors refuse to take it seriously and consider it to be just a minor irritation?

My uncertainty about the future spilled over into my conversations with Lowell. Lowell and I were already having disagreements about how much start-up money we needed. He wanted to spend enough money to ensure a great first edition. I was beginning to worry about every cent we were spending. Would I ever be able to pay that back? Was I just going to lose his money and probably his friendship, which I valued more than the money itself? But, in my heart, I knew it wasn't money I worried about. It was my health.

Granted, I had good days and bad days and probably more good than bad. But what would I do on a bad day when I had to appease an unhappy customer? What if I had fibro fog on the day my magazine was going to print? In many jobs outside of journalism, on a bad day, your boss snaps at you, your lunch hour is delayed, or your computer is down for an hour. Bad days in journalism are much worse. On a bad day for an editor, you have fifteen minutes to rewrite a story and place it on a page, knowing that because the story is controversial, attorneys are going to be scrutinizing every word and looking for a lawsuit. You have to fact-check something while the foreman from the pressroom is shrieking at you because you are missing deadline. You have a photographer who comes back with a camera full of blurred images that you desperately need for that front page. You can't have a bad day when you aren't at your best.

Simply put, I was losing my nerve. I had gotten better, but I had reached a plateau. I couldn't say I was still improving. The chronic pain and lack of sleep still made me difficult to deal with. How much smiling and schmoozing could I do when I could hardly walk?

All my life, when I envisioned myself as a business owner, I saw myself at the Chamber of Commerce, giving speeches and shaking hands. It wasn't my favorite thing to do actually. I prefer a quiet room and a good book. But it was something I could do, and the idea of getting rewarded for my talent and effort without having to support a boss, his boss, and three other upper-management overlords was tempting, if I could do it at all.

Most chronically ill people suffer from what I call the ping-pong syndrome. One day, you're on one side of the optimistic net. Next day, you are on another. One morning, you wake up feeling pretty good, not well, but good. You get up and spend a few minutes trying to decide if this is going to last. And it sometimes does. You're ready to tackle a list of chores. In fact, you've never felt so happy about chores. Every day, you've noted the dust on the end tables, the dirty windows, and the shower stall that so desperately needs a good scrubbing and thought to yourself, "If only ..."

So when a good day dawned, I typically immersed myself in something too large for me to tackle. I started to clean the garage, got half the boxes moved out to the center where I usually parked my car, and then realized that I didn't have the energy to put everything away.

"Well, maybe tomorrow I'll finish this," I told myself.

But I would wake up in pain the next day. It was really more accurate to say the pain woke me up, often much earlier than I normally get up, say 5:00 AM. And this was after the nightly spell from 1:00 to 3:00 when I had no sleep at all. And I was worse than usual, just about as much as I was better yesterday.

There seems to be a forty-eight-hour cycle that is part of our biorhythm. My mother, who suffered from emphysema and rheumatoid arthritis, had forty-eight-hour energy cycles as well, even when she was bedridden.

But when Kevin insisted I work for someone else for awhile before branching out on my own, I turned to Maureen, my acupuncturist. She thought I would be a great business owner. But what was wrong with putting off a new business for a year or so and working for someone else while I proved that I could handle a full-time job? She said the opportunity to open a business would still be there. I could sharpen my skills and get back into a regular routine.

She made sense. What Kevin was saying made sense. I still wanted to go it alone, and everything in my heart said I could, but my health

---

"I Have FMS, and I Work Full-time."

Because the severity of fibromyalgia varies so much from patient to patient, don't compare yourself to others, and don't let your friends do it either. They will often be confused because they heard that someone else they know has FMS and is still working. It's hard for them to understand that some of us have more severe symptoms than others. After all, even with a common cold, symptoms vary in intensity. According to estimates, 20 percent of FMS sufferers can hold a job. Don't feel like a malingerer if you find you can't work. Keep in mind that many doctors apply the label "fibromyalgia" to everything from menstrual cramps to arthritis, so many people who claim to have FMS actually don't.

was the one factor I couldn't seem to control. Reluctantly, I sent an application to the *Reno Gazette-Journal* and another small paper in the area. I could tackle the world later. Or so I thought. Within the next month, I had not one job offer, but two, as both papers courted me.

As luck would have it (or decidedly not), I interviewed for both jobs in the same week. Between interviews, I hit the racks at Macy's. I had put on weight since my last real job. It's amazing what ten pounds does when you are five-foot-two. I had gone from a size six/eight to a size eight/ten, not an unusual weight gain considering I had gone through menopause. But I felt enormously guilty about it and blamed myself because some health professionals believe that weight gain and lack of exercise contribute to FMS. A few even hint that obesity and lack of muscle tone might in fact be the sole cause of FMS. A chiropractor I visited (once and only once) had told me that flat out, "You go down to the gym, get a membership, and try swimming a couple days a week. When you're really out of shape, everything you do causes pain."

Looking at his potbelly and oversized chin, I was in a lot better shape than he was. I was only ten pounds overweight, and that was by my own standards. By most charts, I was still within the normal range, albeit at the high end. He clearly was not in normal range, but he was a man lucky enough to be in good health, which I guess gave him the right to insult me.

But he was not alone in thinking that fibromyalgia is the result of flabby, underused muscles. Maybe he had been reading *Reversing Fibromyalgia*, which postulates:

It's also been suggested that fibromyalgia pain is related to micro trauma in deconditioned muscles, and that the right kind of exercise is beneficial for reconditioning those muscles.

In addition to being out-of-shape, most so-called fibro experts assume all FMS patients are fat. In *Fibromyalgia: A Comprehensive Approach*, author Miryam Ehrlich Williamson describes us, "You look healthy, in an overweight kind of way."

Granted, there were times when I did hurt too much to exercise and when chocolate cake was more welcome than the strongest pain reliever, but weight gain happens to some FMS patients even when they eat less than they have before, perhaps because of an underlying thyroid disorder. And not all FMS patients are overweight. I have met some who were thin as a rail. Certainly, most of the antidepressants we take, sometimes two or three at a time, can cause weight gain. Dr. Rhoades also pointed out that he has never seen a single study that proves or even suggests that weight loss has reduced symptoms in chronic pain patients.

They call FMS a syndrome, a collection of symptoms, instead of a disease like Parkinson's. And it does seem to me to be a syndrome in the sense that it attracts more and more punishment. It's not enough just to have pain, sleeplessness, and forgetfulness. Pretty soon, you're labeled as fat, lazy, unmotivated, depressed, and stupid as well. And this comes from doctors and health practitioners, the very people who are supposed to be helping you!

In any event, my weight gain gave me an excuse to buy new clothes. Because I had been exercising frequently, I still looked pretty good in them. As much as I had enjoyed sitting around in my pajamas, getting dressed up made me feel like a professional again.

I have never felt more victorious than I did that week. I performed on those interviews like I had never performed before. I felt like a prisoner whose sentence had been commuted. I felt terrific. My pain level was below a five. I even slept better than usual. This could have been quite by chance, as my comfort level rose and fell day by day and week by week, or it could have been at my elation that, after three years out of journalism, I was still a hot property. Both of my prospective employers asked me right away if I were interviewing somewhere else, and I could tell they were rushing through the interview process to get their offer in first.

I felt like I had been sitting at a red light for years, and now the signal was go, go, go. I refused to entertain any negative thoughts. I paid less attention to my aches and pains. If I was exhausted at night, it was because I was adjusting to my new life. I had also decided to tell both prospective employers that I had fibromyalgia. Maureen and I didn't agree on this. She didn't feel I needed to apprise anyone in my professional circle of my situation.

But I knew I would be very angry if I hired someone, only to be told three months into the job, that I was now going on disability because of a medical condition I didn't know about. But, all things considered, most of all, I wanted to protect my professional reputation. I wanted to be able to say without hesitation that I had integrity.

Not to worry. When I said I had fibromyalgia, I might as well have been confessing to clogged nasal passages. No one asked a single question, not even when I stressed that the one thing I could not do was sit at a computer all day long. Because these were editing positions, I would be attending meetings and have other responsibilities besides editing copy. In retrospect, I guess I shouldn't have been surprised at their ignorance and nonchalance. How could I expect my potential bosses to be alarmed at the prospect of hiring someone with fibromyalgia when, because of my own lack of knowledge, I hadn't even been overly concerned when I was diagnosed with it? Later, of course, when I couldn't do what they had expected, telling the truth up front couldn't save me from failure. You can't modify a job so an employee can sit in a hot tub of water for hours on end or switch positions, from sitting to standing to walking to stretching to lying down, every ten or fifteen minutes. You can't ask an employer to forgive your forgetfulness when you've forgotten an important assignment. If you're mentally and physically disabled, there's sometimes no amount of accommodations, reasonable or otherwise, to ensure your success.

But before I accepted the job in Reno and started working there, I couldn't have foreseen what would happen. In fact, I would have bet my life that I was returning to a successful career. I did bet my life on it. I thought I could be more than a features editor, but maybe a managing editor at a large metro someday. Maybe I'd get that Pulitzer I'd always dreamed of.

My sister, who had suffered from fibromyalgia for years, tried to warn me that remission could last for months or maybe even a year. But I didn't really hear her. I thought about all the money I had spent on acupuncture, all the days I spent lying in bed while reading Jane Austen and resting and how it had all paid off. I remembered the previous year when I had tried out for the job as part-time editor and hadn't been able to work a full day. I felt victorious just for getting through the week. My body hadn't let me down. It felt better than any award I had ever received, commendation, compliment, or bonus. It felt better than when I drove home my first brand-new company car.

I had three weeks before I started my new job, and I spent them cleaning the garage and deep-cleaning the house in preparation for my new work schedule. My pain remained at an all-time low. I went to aerobics three or four times a week.

"You can conquer fibromyalgia," I told myself.

You can't cure it, but you can reverse it. I fully believed what I had read in the dozen or so fibro bibles, now highlighted and dog-eared on my bookshelf. I believed what the doctors and health practitioners had told me. I was ready to write my own success story.

It was a good thing I waited because, four months later, I was ready to kill myself.

Massage has so many benefits for people with FM; it's just incredible.

Alternative Treatments for Fibromyalgia
and Chronic Fatigue Syndrome

Chapter Ten

The Charm School of Massage

Private offices in the newspaper business are hard to come by. My office at the *Reno Gazette-Journal* was larger than Lou Grant's and more attractive as well. It had a large window facing the lawn, plenty of built-in drawers and cabinets, and a huge desk. But it could have been a broom closet with overflowing waste baskets, and I wouldn't have cared. I thought the first week went well. On Thursday afternoon, I left early for my acupuncture appointment, and I didn't feel at all shy about telling my boss. I was thankful I had told her about my illness. It made things so much easier.

I went right from work to Maureen's office. It was the first time she had ever seen me dressed up. In the waiting room, I glanced through the paper and noticed for the first time that my name was on the front page of the features section, Linda Meilink, features editor. I carried it with me into Maureen's office.

"Working girl," she said approvingly as I walked in, giving me a you-go-girl smile.

I handed her the paper, and we both admired it.

But when the weekend came, I didn't feel so well. I didn't really expect to. I was exhausted and didn't seem to recover. I didn't even do chores.

My second week was even more painful. I had to work late one night, and I didn't seem to catch up the rest of the week. On the weekend, I was of two minds. One said, "Gee, my house is really dirty." The other

---

House Calls

Keeping up with housework is a problem if you can hardly hold a broom. Enlist family when you can. Hire professionals. Also very helpful is the book, *Clean Your House the Lazy Way* by Barbara Durham.

---

one said, "You can't possibly do this housework. You can hardly walk. Are you out of your mind?"

Instead of sitting down calmly and explaining the problem to Kevin, I had a temper tantrum. I didn't want to tell him I needed help and lots of it. Instead, I complained he wasn't doing his share of the housework. Well, he wasn't, but I wasn't either.

The house was becoming more and more squalid. Kevin occasionally helped by sweeping the floors or throwing a few loads of clothes into the washing machine, but his idea of cleanliness and mine were more like antonyms than synonyms. The bathrooms went unscrubbed, and the sheets went unchanged. Dog hair began to cover our couch. The house was filthy, filthy, filthy. I yelled at him for not using a coaster, not picking up his socks, and leaving laundry in the drier instead of folding it and putting it away. After one of my sullen outbursts, Kevin, God bless him, saw through my hysteria and realized I was too sick to help with the housework.

"Tell me what to do, and I will do it," he said. "Make a list and I'll do all the housework."

He picked up a broom and bucket. Every night after that, I came home to a tidy and dust-free house.

By the third week, the pain was more pronounced. Hell, it wasn't just pronounced. It was speaking to me with a French accent. My lower back hurt so bad that I started standing up to type at work. Some days, I lowered the blinds in my office, locked the door, lay down on the floor, grasped my ankles, and pulled them over my head, trying to stretch out the muscle spasms in my lower back. My boss came by one day and opened my blinds. I realized no other managers had their blinds closed. Obviously having my own office didn't translate into any real privacy.

As the weeks went on and I became more exhausted, my responsibilities at work increased. I came in earlier, trying to get a head start, but never managed to leave on time.

I began to skip my acupuncture appointments. Maureen had moved from Reno to Carson City, nearly an hourlong drive each way. It was irrational of me, but I felt betrayed by the move. It was painful to make the long drive after sitting at a computer. In the beginning, I thought it was the poor design of car seats, but, even when I was lying in the backseat while Kevin drove, riding was still horrendously painful on bad days. I think it may be the vibration of the car on a fragile and overexcited nervous system.

So while acupuncture still brought down my pain level, I could hardly make the drive there to get it. And the benefit had sometimes worn off before I got home.

I did begin to appreciate the benefits of massage. I would occasionally slip away from work at a decent hour and get a full-body massage at a spa close to my home. But it would be only a few hours before the all-too-familiar muscle pains would snap back.

With a full-time job, I couldn't nap in the afternoon if I needed to. On top of the wrenching pain, I was exhausted from lack of sleep. I went to my family doctor, who prescribed sleeping pills. I

Grin and Bear It

The National Center of Health Statistics Report concluded that chronic pain patients today are more apt to go to work rather than call in sick.

knew they were addictive, and I had previously limited them to one night a week, usually Sunday night because Mondays were always the most stressful days for me. Now I no longer cared that they were addictive. I needed to sleep at all costs.

I called my younger sister, Suzie, for help. She had learned to balance a demanding and successful career with disabling asthma, arthritis, and a host of other health problems.

"What can I do?" I asked her. "I desperately want to keep this job."

"Do what you have to do," she said. "Take breaks. Go out to lunch. Tell your boss."

"I can't tell my boss," I said. "I'm afraid to. I'm still on probation."

"Then do whatever you have to do. Get a massage every day if you need to."

I began to get massages two or three times a week. Then something strange started to happen. The massages seemed to aggravate rather than alleviate my symptoms. I can't blame it on masseuses because I went to the same ones I always had. My disease was progressing to the point where it hurt to be touched. Even light massage could be painful. And I'd sometimes leave my session feeling a bit better, only to find that, an hour later, I felt much worse than I had before the massage.

Most fibromyalgia experts highly recommend massage. According to *Chronic Fatigue Syndrome, Fibromyalgia and other Invisible Symptoms* by Katrina Berne, PhD:

> Massotherapy, or massage, offers a multitude of benefits: pain relief, increased circulation, removal of toxins from the body, "unlocking" tight muscles, and encouraging relaxation. Types of massage include Swedish massage for relaxation; myofascial massage, deep-tissue work to relieve pain and tightness; reflexology, the stimulation of points on the hands and feet that correspond to body organs; and shiatsu, the application of strong pressure to points along meridians corresponding to lymph channels, often painful but ultimately relaxing.

I have tried all of these different types of massage. When my symptoms were mild to moderate, they worked very well. I eventually taught some of the most helpful techniques to Kevin. A quick rub from him for ten to twenty minutes is not only less expensive, but it is more effective because he knows just where to go, depending on where the pain is greatest.

At a Web site where patients rate their responses to various treatments, massage is rated at a seven-point effectiveness on a scale of ten. Most of the comments are positive. A few complain that the massage actually seemed to make them worse. As of the date I am writing, massage is rated nearly one point higher than acupuncture. I can't stress enough that the effectiveness of these treatments varies from patient to patient, and there is nothing wrong with trying all of them. Just remember that a successful treatment will go a long way in alleviating your symptoms, but it may not work for you. You should immediately stop any therapy that seems to be irritating you, even if your masseuse or other practitioner encourages you to continue. One time while my sister was working with a physical therapist to relieve her fibromyalgia symptoms, he encouraged her to walk up and down steps, which led to a strained ankle, a cast, and six months of agony. No one knows your body like you, so be wary. Therapists are often deceived about your level or pain because, as everyone tells you that you "look okay."

The biggest complaint about massage is that it is expensive, generally $60 to $70 a session, and insurance often does not cover it. This is changing though, so you might ask your doctor for a prescription for massages.

When I was working, I figured it didn't matter if I spent a third of my income on massage because, without it, I might not be working at all. You have to schedule them in advance, however. With my work schedule, that was sometimes a problem.

Once, in desperation, I called one at random in the phone book under "Massage-therapeutic." They booked me in that same night. The waiting area looked a bit like a storefront rather than a spa. There were no chairs, just a few shelves stocked with health products. A skinny, bespectacled man stood behind the cash register. He smiled broadly when I said I had an appointment. Instead of asking me to fill out a form disclosing any physical maladies, he asked me to pay in advance. And he wouldn't take my credit card. He pointed out an ATM machine outside a casino across the street. I ran over there to pump out $80 in cash, $60 for the massage and something extra for a tip.

I was ushered upstairs immediately. As I followed my therapist up the stairs, I noted she had on a flowered print dress and moderately high heels, no white nurse shoes for this girl. She had curly blonde hair that extended below her shoulders. It was evident she had spent her share of time at make-up counters and had probably gotten some bad advice at them, too.

But I didn't care. I could hardly walk up the stairs. I wanted a massage, and I wanted it now. I limped up the steep, wooden stairs and into the tiny room. I got undressed and stretched out on the clean, white cot. Should I have guessed what was going on when I smelled her perfume? Massage therapists don't wear perfume. It irritates patients with chemical sensitivity disorders.

And I might have guessed something was amiss if I had been a bit more clear-headed, but I hurt like a bicyclist who has just driven off a cliff. My perceptions were so murky and confused that I felt like I was on a San Francisco wharf as the dense fog comes rolling in. I'm a journalist, and I'm usually always suspicious, but I didn't catch on, not even after she came in quietly and started stroking my back, lightly running her fingertips up and down my spine.

"You can rub harder than that," I suggested.

The pressure increased, but the caress didn't stop. Then she leaned across me. I could feel her hair brush across my shoulder.

"If you want anything special," she whispered huskily, "just ask."

Okay, so now I got it. Well, there was also one other clue. She had liquor on her breath. I lay very still. I was afraid she would take any movement on my part as an invitation. By now, she had branched out, her fingers trailing up and down my arms. Embarrassed? Yeah, a bit. Anxious? A little. But I was actually in so much pain that all I felt was disappointment. I wanted to cry. I wanted my massage, and this wasn't getting it. Then, as she leaned over, a piece of her jewelry got caught in the sheet.

"Sorry," she said as she untangled herself.

I began to feel sorry for her. She seemed as confused as I was. How do you proposition a woman as old as your mother? As a journalist, I had always wanted to interview a professional sex therapist. Despite my pain, misery, and general discomfort, I didn't want to miss my chance.

"What made you decide to become a masseuse?" I asked.

She giggled. I could tell she was a bit drunk. "Well, I used to work across the street at the casino as a cocktail waitress. One day, my boss called me in and said, 'You're too good to be doing this.' And so he promoted me to masseuse."

"Where did you go to school?"

"Oh, I take classes," she said. "I take classes all the time."

"Do you like it?" I asked.

"Oh, yes," she said sincerely. "I like to make people happy. That's just who I am, I guess. Lots of people in the world today don't care, but I do. I really care. Are you sure you don't want anything special?"

I thanked her. After all, no matter who she was, there was no reason for me not to have good manners. And I tipped her, although clearly less than what she had hoped to earn. I went downstairs where the glassy-eyed clerk leered at me. You could tell he had some powerful fantasies. I could see myself in the mirror on the back wall with my hair tousled and my face pink.

So here's one more piece of advice you won't hear in the typical fibromyalgia support group. Get a reference for a masseuse. Unless you're up for something more thrilling than a back rub (and if you are), God bless you. You have something most of us don't have, a sex drive.

And no matter what ridiculous things you have done to make yourself feel better, remember that you probably have better judgment than I do. You probably never paid a hooker and got nothing out of it.

All achievement and success that is meaningful has its beginning with desire and is brought to fruition only if one believes strongly enough that it will happen.

Joe Elrod, *Reversing Fibromyalgia*

Chapter Eleven

The Painful Price of Perseverance

That great job, the one with the office, the nice salary, the nameplate, and the opportunity to do things I loved to do, nearly killed me. And all the positive thinking, reading, proselytizing, and cheerleading by my doctors, massage therapists, chiropractors, and authors of self-help books were accomplices.

From the third week on, there was no let up in the pain. It was an act of heroism to drive home every night. I could hardly hold the steering wheel. Once home, I'd sit in the chair, no longer able to concentrate on television. I'd watch the clock, waiting for 8:00 PM when I could take the prescription sleeping medicine that had become a nightly ritual and knock myself out. I'd lie there, feeling the pain subside only slightly before I fell into a trance.

The pain was like a fire from which there was no escape, not for a minute or a second. It woke me up every morning. I had to get in the bathtub to loosen up so I could get dressed. So why didn't I quit my job?

In fact, the worse the pain got, the less I thought about quitting my job. I really couldn't make a decision anymore. I was totally insane. I had spent years working, doing everything I was supposed to do, exercising, eating celery, meditating, walking, and thinking lovely thoughts about sailboats off the coast of San Diego. My determination at this point was deeper than the worst imaginable pain. As long as I could put one foot in front of the other, I told myself, "I'm going to go to work."

Taking a Break

The Family Medical Leave Act (FMLA) allows chronic pain patients to take up to twelve months. However, to qualify, you must have been employed by your company for at least a year, and your company must have at least fifty employees.

I don't remember a lot about those four months. It's natural to have amnesia and confusion when you are in extreme pain. The brain can only handle so much. One day at an editorial meeting, someone asked me what was going to run in my section the next day, and I couldn't remember. I couldn't even speak. The whole room hummed with silence. Everyone stared at me.

I finally croaked out, "I don't remember."

My boss said kindly, "Well, that happens to all of us sometimes," but she was lying.

No one else ever forgot something that important, especially when we were going to that meeting expressly to talk about the next day's paper. After that, I never went to a meeting without a cheat sheet in which I had written down any details I thought I might be quizzed on.

I found the easiest way to stay out of trouble was to prattle along with feigned enthusiasm as I recited the next day's stories. It made me look like something of a bubblehead, but an inoffensive bubblehead. Instead of wanting to impress my bosses, I just wanted to stay out of their way. There was once a time when I couldn't get enough attention. I loved heated newsroom debates and invigorating discussions with my boss over lunch.

Now all I wanted was to keep my head down and get along because I couldn't cope with anything else. The only doctor I consulted was my family physician, who prescribed nightly sleeping medication. She had referred me to a pain doctor, but the paperwork was somehow never approved. Whenever I called the specialist's office, they'd refer me back to my doctor. I thought maybe Ambien, a popular sleeping pill, would fix everything. I slept deeply, but the pain was even deeper. At work, during lengthy meetings, I started bringing a stuffed pillow that I heated up in the microwave.

"Does that really help?" my boss asked once pointedly.

I was embarrassed, as if I were bringing it along as a prop to get attention or advertise my condition, but I could barely sit without it. I tried to get to meetings early so I could sit in one of the padded chairs. Those who came at the last minute were relegated to wooden chairs along the wall. Even worse were the metal folding chairs we sat in at monthly staff meetings.

Then I had two female employees with similar, unusual names: Siobhan and Sevil. I couldn't get their names straight.

"Who's doing the back-to-school story?" my boss would ask.

"Siobhan," I would answer.

"I thought Sevil was doing it."

"Oh, that's right. Sevil is doing it."

I explained to her one day that I sometimes substituted one word for another. It was part of the fibromyalgia syndrome. I was trying to assure her that I really did know what was going on and who was in charge of which story. But, truthfully, on some days, I didn't know. And I know she knew.

On top of my problems at work and problems with my husband, I also argued with my acupuncturist, Maureen, something that hadn't happened before. I no longer kept regular appointments because the drive was excruciating. I limped into her office, barely able to climb on the table. At first, she simply advised me to cut back on hours, eat better, and rest more, but I could soon tell that she didn't like what was happening to me.

Migraine Connection

Researchers have noted that fibromyalgia and migraine share many of the same triggers. Some of these triggers are bright lights, change in weather, and lack of sleep. Some sufferers of both conditions report a feeling of energy and well-being before a flare-up begins.

Once when I drove up for an emergency acupuncture session, she asked about my diet and exercising. I don't know what I answered, but I know it was testy because I remember her saying, "You sure have changed since you started working."

"I'm not telling you to quit your job," she said at my next visit.

And she didn't. Not yet. But we both knew I couldn't do what she was asking me to do, eat right, exercise, keep regular appointments, and still work full-time in my current position.

One day after my acupuncture, I had such a severe muscle spasm that I couldn't get off the table. She had to apply lengthy acupressure to release the contraction in my back so I could get up.

I didn't want to tell Kevin that I was falling apart. He was doing everything he could to help me. He was overjoyed I had gone back to work. When I first started, he had confided that he was secretly worried about what would have happened if I couldn't work and he had to be financially responsible for both of us forever. I later knew he was sorry he had said it, and I know I was. I liked to believe that it didn't really make much difference to him if I worked or not. I wanted to think that he liked having me at home, folding his T-shirts and cooking some Thai curry, even if I really couldn't do much cooking and cleaning.

Now I knew how much he wanted me to work, and I didn't want to let him down. I didn't want to go back to living on his salary. I liked spending more money, and I particularly like spending my own money. I wanted to go back to Europe someday, traipse through the Far East (Cambodia, Thailand, and Malaysia), and wander through Africa and watch elephants in the wild. But in the meantime, I had to worry about driving to work safely.

Even though I had told my boss when I was hired that I couldn't spend lengthy hours at the computer, somehow that was forgotten after I started. I was supposed to be learning a new computer system. I used to be pretty good at picking up new journalism software systems, but this time I struggled, making the same mistakes over and over, writing notes and losing them, or being unable to understand them. My boss told me I would have to fill in for some staff on the computer during Christmas vacations, and I couldn't imagine how I could do it when an hour or so was crippling. And that wasn't the worst of it. The worst was that I couldn't seem to learn it.

Instead of getting shorter, my days got longer. My responsibilities continued to increase. I was now coming in Saturdays for a few hours to work on the computer. Two weeks before Thanksgiving, I had an incredibly long to-do list, including three personnel evaluations. I asked if I could turn one in late. Nothing doing. It was clear that whatever accommodations they were willing to make for my health condition did not include a reduction of responsibilities.

Mornings were the worst. At night, I'd sit with my sleeping pills in my hand, wondering how many it would take to put me to sleep permanently. I didn't want to die. I just didn't want to wake up in pain anymore. Even the recognition that I was suicidal didn't stop me from wanting to keep that job because I wanted the money. I wanted the responsibilities, even though they were too much for me. I wanted to stay in journalism, no matter what it cost and how bad this particular job was.

I still liked editing stories and working with reporters, writing headlines, and proofing pages. I had spent the last few years as an outsider looking in, and I didn't want to go back to sitting at home reading the daily news, feeling bitter and resentful because I knew I could have written a better story, found an error, or written a catchier headline.

Kevin was worried. When he was close enough to overhear me in the newsroom, even my voice didn't sound the same.

He said, "When I look up and see you, you're white as a ghost, and you look like a zombie."

I kept thinking that, if I kept doing the same thing repeatedly each day, my body would eventually adjust. It's like the story of the thrifty farmer who starved his horse to death by trying to cure him of eating.

In the middle of November, I managed to break away to get my annual Pap smear, which was already a year overdue. I was annoyed at having to keep the appointment, and I sat in the examining room editing some work I had brought with me when the doctor came in.

The first thing she said to me was, "Your blood pressure is 180 over 120. What is going on?"

Nothing was going on that hadn't been going on. I had been telling her about the pain for months. But she hadn't seemed to pay much attention until it was driving up my blood pressure.

"You can't go back to work," she said as she scribbled some prescriptions. "You have to go home and rest."

"I have to go back to work. I have a meeting in an hour."

"I'll give you a note."

Hate to Exercise?

Most of us hate sit-ups, push-ups, and boring workouts, but there are many other ways to get some light exercise while enjoying yourself. If you can't bear water aerobics, Tai Chi, or walking, here are some activities that will get your blood flowing:

Miniature golf
Ping-pong
Croquet
Bicycling
Ballroom dancing
Darts
Shuffleboard
Pool
Light gardening
Sex
Yoga
Tap dancing

"I don't want a note. I don't want anyone to know."

"Are you listening to me? You're going to have a stroke. You have to go home and lie down. You need to take at least two weeks off."

"I can't take off two weeks. My staff is going on vacation over Thanksgiving."

In the end, she gave up and handed me prescriptions for blood pressure medication, more pain pills, a muscle relaxant, and Cymbalta, even though I told her I never wanted to take antidepressants again. I shoved the prescriptions into my purse, drove back to work, and called Kevin. He was just getting ready to leave for work.

I didn't bother to go into details about the doctor's appointment. I just told him to come over right now and bring my Valium. As soon as he came in, I took ten milligrams, twice my usual dose, and went to the meeting. I worked the rest of the week and stayed in bed all weekend. Hot baths, cold packs, painkillers, muscle relaxants, and stretching exercises, nothing stopped the pain. It was a huge, blinding white fire. I could barely get out of bed. It hurt to walk. It hurt to lie still.

On Monday, I went back to work. I was beaten, and I knew it, but I wouldn't give up. I went through the motions as best I could, waiting for some let-up in the pain. There was none. It took everything I had to walk across the parking lot at the end of the day and drive home.

Getting caught by a red light was a nightmare because it meant one or two minutes longer before I could get into a hot bath or try another pill, although none of them were working. The only one I hadn't tried yet was the antidepressant.

Thursday was Thanksgiving, and Kevin had to work. We met some of his co-workers downtown for an early dinner. I hurt so badly that I could hardly sit up. After we finished dinner, as the rest of our party filed out the door, I went into the bathroom and threw up.

On Friday morning, I went back to work. I had promised to help the assistant features editor with some computer work. I wasn't much

---

Myofascial Pain

Myofascial pain is caused by muscle spasms that are felt as hard lumps under the skin. These are not the same as trigger-point discomfort. These knots feel like hard rocks that sometimes seem to move or spread from one part of the body to another. They can often be relieved somewhat by hot and/or cold packs, massage, acupuncture and acupressure.

help, but I insisted on staying until the pages went out about 7:00 PM. As Kevin walked me out of the building, I knew I was not coming back. I knew this was my last day.

All night long, the pain continued to spike. I thought, as I often had, about going to the emergency room, but I somehow made it through. The next morning, I put all my medications in a plastic bag. I must have had prescriptions for about fifteen or twenty drugs at this point, and Kevin drove me to see Maureen. When she came in the room, I started to cry and couldn't stop. For the first time, I talked about not really wanting to live anymore because the pain was so severe. I didn't want to die. I just wanted the pain to end.

She listened as Kevin and I both talked. She talked to me about wanting to keep my job; she talked to Kevin about what was happening to me. She listed all the drugs I had been taking. Then she deftly inserted the needles. My body was so conditioned to acupuncture that I could feel myself relax as soon as the first needles went in. She left us in a dark-ened room for about forty minutes. Kevin dozed in a chair in the corner of my room during the treatment. The pain went down a notch or two.

When it was over, she came in and sat down. "I'm not telling you that you won't ever be able to go back to work, but you need at least six weeks of rest. And then we'll have to reevaluate."

Six weeks? I was fretting over two weeks. As for the pain relievers, she had once told me not to take them, but she wouldn't say that anymore.

"You sometimes need them," she said. "We both thought you were ready to go back to work. It didn't hurt to try, but it just doesn't look like this is working out."

I was still argumentative and incredulous. Surely something could be done besides resigning? In an effort to show me how badly my condition had deteriorated, she read to us from her progress notes from the previous year.

"Reports pain level significantly lower. Has increased energy."

"Exercising four times a week."

"Teaching classes and sleeping better. Less pain."

Then she read from her chart since I had started work. That finally broke through my denial.

I went home, rested, and called my sisters. They commiserated with me, but agreed with Maureen. I sobbed all weekend. Late Sunday afternoon, I began to feel a bit better. I told my older sister I changed my mind. I was going back the next day.

"Just to see how I do," I said.

Ten minutes after we hung up, my younger sister called. She was blunt and to the point. "Darlene says you're going back to work tomorrow."

She is the younger sister, but she has a bossy streak. I could tell she was pitched for a battle.

"Don't worry. I've already changed my mind."

And it was true. Whatever fleeting relief I had felt was already gone. I called in sick the next day, stayed home, and waited for the pain to go away, but, if anything, it got worse. A week went by and then two. I called in sick every day. I went back to my family doctor, who seemed exasperated when I told her I felt hopeless and unable to tolerate the pain anymore. I hadn't tried the antidepressants either.

The sympathy she had once felt for me was exhausted. My complaints, fears, and distress clearly annoyed her.

"You've got to change your attitude," she said, her anger evident in her tone. "You won't get well if you don't think positive."

Okay, so I tried to think positive when I woke up in the morning and wondered if I could move my arms and legs enough to roll out of bed. I tried to think positive as I walked around the house in slow motion because it hurt to stand up and it hurt to sit down. I tried to think positive as I watched my career slip away. And I tried to think positive as I downed a handful of pills every morning.

I was glad my husband had been in the room with the doctor and me. Even after everything I had told him about my doctors, her tone surprised him.

"I thought you were seeing a pain specialist," she said accusingly, as if I were neglecting my problems.

"I keep calling for an appointment, but they never call me back."

To her credit, she must have pulled some strings, because, within a day or two, I got a call from a pain doctor who was able to get me an appointment right away. Then things started to happen. I liked the pain specialist immediately. Pain specialists are different than GPs. They don't expect you to get better. They know you are there because no other treatment has worked. Their job is try to make you comfortable, whether you are dying of cancer or just incapacitated by a bad back.

As for my job, the pain doctor was brutally direct. I could not continue what I was doing.

"I'm not saying that, at some time in the future, you may not be able to work part-time," she said.

But pressuring myself to perform, work, and will myself to be well was destroying me. Enduring wracking pain was doing my body more harm than any pain medicine or tranquilizer would do. For example, chronic pain can make a driver just as incompetent as one who is woozy on drugs, although neither is in a condition to be driving. Pain gave me a terrific case of road rage. It made me take chances I wouldn't have taken before, like rushing through a light as it changed to red so I could get home a few seconds earlier and get in a hot bath. I swore at drivers who dawdled and passed them on the right. I drove too fast. I could have gladly driven over an elderly jaywalker if it cut a few minutes from my trip. I was, in fact, a much better driver with a few milligrams of Valium in my system.

She was the first doctor who explained to me how pain alone could debilitate your mind and body, that is, how it causes your neurons to misfire, leaving you confused and disoriented.

"The brain can only take so much," she said. "And then it misfires. It begins to short-circuit."

Pain also creates a cycle. The more pain, the more the muscles and other tissues tighten up and go into spasm, creating more pain, which causes more tightening. Pain medications can stop those cycles and even prevent them from happening.

Part-time Perks

Most of us believe you have to choose between Social Security disability and working, but it's not necessarily so. You can work part-time and keep what you earn up to a certain limit without losing your SSI.

Instead of waiting until the pain was nearly unbearable, she wanted me to take pain medicine on a regular cycle to keep the pain from spiking.

She was the first medical doctor I had ever talked to who understood what I was going through. As for my blood pressure, the nausea, dizziness, and other symptoms, they were most likely a response to elevated pain.

She said there was a list of pain relievers we could try. And we would have to try several before we found the right one. She felt sure that, someday in the relatively near future, doctors would learn how to treat fibromyalgia. The trick was keeping the patients alive long enough.

I wasn't sure I wanted to live that long, not with that kind of pain and not for ten years. Not even five. Sometimes, not even one day.

I didn't realize the pain relief I was resisting would end up being a lifesaver. I was biased against pain medicine because so many doctors had told me to avoid it, so I only took it when I was at the breaking point. From her, I learned not to wait until I suffered unbearable pain before I took an anesthetic of one sort or another. Both Vicodin and OxyContin work well for me; other pain medicines and antidepressants haven't worked as well. But because of my ignorance and the ignorance of my doctors, I had spent years before I found someone who was willing to teach me how to deal with pain. Most of my doctors had advised against taking anything stronger than Motrin.

Fortunately, many doctors are beginning to speak up about the need for stronger pain meds for fibromyalgia patients. In the foreword to *Alternative Treatments for Fibromyalgia & Chronic Pain Syndrome*, Dr. Paul Brown, a fibromyalgia specialist in Seattle, wrote:

> Patients with other diseases that cause chronic pain are given narcotic analgesics if they don't respond to less potent pain relievers. The same should be true for FMS patients, but this is not always the case. Treatment with narcotics, when necessary, can alleviate the pain, fatigue, and cognitive problems, permitting patients to feel and function better.

Arthur Rosenfeld, in *The Truth about Chronic Pain*, was even stronger in his discussion on how debilitating chronic pain can be:

> As recently as 15 years ago, doctors were still performing surgery on infants without anesthesia, using only paralytic agents to make sure they didn't move. Many circumcisions are still performed without anesthesia, even though tests now show that fetuses as young as 23 weeks respond to painful stimuli. Doctors now know that pain interferes with recovery; that it hampers an organism's ability to heal; that it brings with it direct physical consequences, such as increased blood pressure and resulting stroke, heart attack, seizure or

brain hemorrhage. Medical researchers have also discovered that untreated pain has the sort of emotional consequences—fears, phobias, delayed defense reactions and sensitivities—in test animals that make one wonder whether the brutalities until recently visited on infants might later in life lead to violent or sociopathic behavior, or a predilection toward substance abuse.

For the next few months, I dutifully swallowed white and yellow, little round pills, capsules, and large oval, evil-tasting drugs that stuck in my throat. We kept looking for something that would work for me without making me ill. Some of them didn't work at all or worked only for short periods. Ultram, for instance, seemed to have no effect at all on me, except that the pain seemed to increase as the pills wore off. Percocet made me hazily indifferent to the pain for the first few days, and then that quit working. Vicodin, while technically less strong than Percocet, had the most reliable results.

I was hopeful I would find the right combination that would leave me relieved but relatively clear-headed. This was when I finally gave in and started taking the antidepressant Cymbalta, which was supposed to relieve pain along with depression. Earlier, Cymbalta had given me such intense withdrawal symptoms that I continue to take it to this day. But, during the first few days on Cymbalta, it was almost as bad as withdrawal. Thanks to the Cymbalta, I threw up all over Tijuana, where I had gone on a day trip with Lowell and his wife, and Kevin.

We started Saturday with a real Mexican breakfast: ranchos huevos, rice, and hot salsa. I love Mexican food, the hotter the better. I thoroughly enjoyed the huge, steaming platters served with mugs of hot coffee. But as we lingered over our coffee, my stomach lurched. I excused myself, went to the bathroom, and threw up … a lot.

After breakfast, we headed for the high-end district of Tijuana, where million-dollar homes perch on the hillsides overlooking the valley. Pretty soon, the roads seemed to spiral out of control. I was so dizzy that I thought I would faint. Then I threw up. I wasn't just slightly ill. I retched and retched. Every time I could lift my head, I looked up at the houses, expecting someone to come running out and yell at me to quit vomiting on their lawn.

Lowell jumped out of the car. I begged him to get back in so he wouldn't see me. I got back in the car and noticed a small spot of vomit on the inside of the car door. Luckily, I had a water bottle with me and was able to quickly wipe it off with a tissue.

"Oh, dear," Lowell's wife, April, said sympathetically. "She's carsick."

"I don't get carsick," I muttered crossly.

And I don't. I don't get seasick either, not when everyone else is hanging over the side of the boat.

We were soon on a straight and narrow highway, heading off to our next landmark, when Lowell stopped to ask directions. It was fortunate for all of us that we stopped when we did. This time, I threw up without any warning whatsoever. If we hadn't been sitting at the curb, I would have thrown up all over the leather seats and pale, immaculate carpet. I threw open the door and stumbled out, vomiting as I went. There were people outside their houses here, but, if people were staring at me, I didn't know because I didn't look up. Lowell, who was already out of the car, came over to try to help me, but, once again, I begged him to leave me alone.

Well, so much for that trip.

Later, as Lowell and I stood waiting for Kevin and April to use the bathroom, Lowell asked me how much of the time I was in pain.

"Every minute, every day," I said.

We were silent for a minute or two.

"Do you know what I hate most?" I said. "It isn't the pain or the sleepless nights. It's the loss of my career, the feeling of being so useless. Sometimes, I feel like my life is over."

He touched my arm, and we fell silent. There wasn't anything to say.

When we got back home, April insisted I lie down. She brought me a cup of tea and a good book. Nothing was so comforting and familiar.

Within a few hours, I walked out of the guest room and dressed for dinner. The nausea was completely gone. We had a wonderful dinner. When we got back, I looked up Cymbalta on the computer. The list of side effects was pretty overwhelming, including nausea, vomiting, dry mouth, constipation, diarrhea, fatigue, blurred vision, insomnia, anxiety, abnormal orgasm, erectile dysfunction, dizziness, sweating, somnolence, tremor, and increased risk of suicide in teenagers. And these were just the common, expected side effects. Twenty percent of those using Cymbalta for the first time experienced nausea; five percent experienced vomiting.

"Well," I thought, "I won't take that anymore."

Once again, I was wrong. I would start taking Cymbalta again a few weeks later, when I was desperate enough to take anything. I'm not sure if it worked or not because it doesn't start working right away, like painkillers do.

I also tried methadone, the same drug given to junkies to keep them off heroin. My pain doctor insisted it was worth a try. She may have sensed that I was giving up. The drugs weren't helping enough to make a difference, and I was resistant to trying stronger doses. Some of them made me feel weird; others didn't work at all. For many chronic pain sufferers, methadone has given them a whole new life. I read all about it on the Internet. Whenever I ran into someone with a chronic pain problem, I asked if he or she had tried it. A few people swore it was the best thing they had ever tried.

"It's not just a drug for junkies," my doctor insisted. "They give it to drug addicts because it keeps their heads clear."

"Read about it," she suggested when she handed me the prescription. "You can fill this or not."

I asked several pharmacists about methadone as well. Some wouldn't comment; a few told me it was a dead end. Patients quickly become immune to it and need to be on ever-increasing doses.

Maureen was particularly opposed to it. "I have patients who are on methadone, and they still hurt."

My youngest son, a naval officer, didn't like the idea either. He told me that military doctors didn't give their strongest pain medications to injured soldiers unless there was no hope left.

"The body just gives up," he said.

My oldest son, who worked for years as a lab tech for Johnson & Johnson and now is an executive there, was less perturbed. "I don't know, Mom. Everyone responds to drugs differently. It might help. It might not."

The pain specialist was more worried about the severe and debilitating pain. "Try the methadone," she urged as she handed me a prescription. "Just take a little bit. Play around with it."

I carried the prescription in my wallet for at least six months before a particularly nasty flare made me so desperate that I would have tried horse manure if it had any analgesic qualities. I was also interested in methadone because it generally has the fewest psychotropic effects. I was fed up with drugs that made me woozy. My dislike of mind-altering drugs has always seemed a bit ironic to me. With all the junkies in the world who wanted nothing more than a free pass to ingest all the drugs they wanted, everything from Valium to OxyContin, why did I have to be the one who didn't enjoy them?

The first few days after I started a small dose of methadone, I thought I had found God. Only I wasn't high. I felt like some major divine-hand-of-God miracle had

Smooth Away Myofascial Pain

If you can't talk your spouse or best friend into taking a massage class, here are a few quick tips about working with myofascial muscle knots. You can apply direct pressure to the sore spot with your thumb until the knot begins to relax. Or you can rub the areas between the knots. This gets the blood flowing away from the painful site. Hot packs and hot baths are also effective.

cured me. The pain was almost completely gone. I felt alert and energetic. I was a bit too sleepy, and I had a headache that came and went, but those seemed to be the only side effects.

Then on the third or fourth day, I was pulling into a parking lot at a church rummage sale when my whole world seemed to change gears. It was like flipping the channel on television. Everything looked different, kind of garish. It was sunny, but too sunny. I saw a large man crossing the lot, and he looked exaggerated, ballooned out, rather like a cartoon. Although there were several open parking spots, I couldn't decide where to park. I couldn't remember why I was there. The only thing I could think of was that I shouldn't be driving. I managed to park the car, get out, and walk around, hoping the effects would wear off in a few minutes. I felt unreal. I guess this is what "tripping" means in drug lingo. I had just landed on another planet, and there were people here, only they didn't know I was somewhere else. They even talked to me.

This sounds more innocuous than it was. I was terrified. I pretended to look at ugly pictures in chipped frames and old, dirty lampshades. I was too afraid to get in my car and drive home. I didn't dare call Kevin, who was home asleep after working late, because he would have been more frightened for me than I was.

After a few minutes, a half hour, or maybe even a week or two, I remembered that methadone is a long-acting drug, and it was pretty unlikely that these strange sensations would wear off in a few minutes. I finally got back in my car and drove home very carefully. Or at least that's how I remember it. In retrospect, I could have been on the wrong side of the road.

So that was it for methadone. One more drug crossed off my list. I was sorry because I have a neighbor who says it has given him so much pain relief that it changed his life.

In the end, I stuck to Vicodin and oxycodone, an OxyContin-based drug, sometimes boosted with Valium or complemented by Motrin. These drugs seem to have the fewest side effects. Although some of these drugs, particularly some antidepressants, did me more harm than good, I think every FMS patient who can tolerate different classes of pain drugs should have the opportunity to try them and choose what works best. Everyone has unique responses. For this reason, each patient needs to try different medications. In no case do I think there is virtue in needless suffering if you can find something that relieves the pain. If your doctor thinks otherwise, then find another doctor.

In *Pain Free 1-2-3*, Dr. Jacob Teitelbaum, a noted fibromyalgia specialist, writes:

> The stress of pain takes a toll on your body that is not healthy. Pain is simply meant to tell you that there's something wrong that you need to pay attention to. Once you do this, the pain is no longer healthy and should be eliminated. I suspect that you get no bonus points in heaven for having suffered through the pain instead of taking the medications needed to be comfortable. I often tell my patients the story about a pious man who lived in Johnstown during the Johnstown flood. The National Guard came into the city and told everyone to evacuate. This man refused to leave, saying that he had faith in God and God would protect him. The floodwaters came, and soon the Coast Guard boat arrived, floating by his second story win-

dow. They beseeched him to climb in the boat and be saved but he refused, once again saying he had faith in God to protect him. Pretty soon he was up on top of the roof, and a helicopter came by and the pilot yelled at him to get in. Once again he refused—and the man drowned. He went to heaven, and God came by. The man was very angry at God and said, "I had full faith in you and you let me drown!" And God said, "What are you talking about? I sent the National Guard, the Coast Guard, and a helicopter!" The medications are like the National Guard, the Coast Guard, and the helicopter. It's OK to use them!

◆   ◆   ◆

As for my career, it took me several days before I called and resigned from my job. Kevin cleared out my desk for me, sparing me the emotional distress of having to go in and bring home my personal dictionary, thesaurus, Associated Press manual, and the pictures of my grandchildren on the bulletin board across from my desk. Thanks to him, I didn't have to lock the office for the last time and hand in my key, saying goodbye to a newsroom for a third, and perhaps final, time.

I still hadn't learned my lesson, however. Just a few weeks after I resigned from my job in Reno, before I had even tried half the drug therapies my doctor recommended, I was back in the doctor's office, trying to convince her and Kevin that I was well enough to take another job. Was I feeling better? Not really. I still crawled around the house or sat huddled up in the reclining chair with a blanket. I hoped that, with bed rest, herbs, acupuncture, massage (the legitimate kind), and some miracle drugs, I'd be back on my feet in a few weeks. Hadn't Maureen said I needed six weeks of rest? I thought two or three might do it for me.

Kevin had been offered a better job in Modesto, and I didn't really have to apply to snag an interview. A former co-worker who now worked at the paper recommended me for a reporting job. When I went up to Modesto to look for a house, I stopped by the newspaper, ostensibly just to meet the editor.

When I told Kevin I might have a job, I really thought he would be happy and relieved. Instead, he looked at me as if I had just told him I had signed up to become an astronaut. Apparently, he and I had heard two very different things from my doctors. I had heard that I could go back to work. He had heard them say I might be able to go back to work someday if I found the right job and worked part-time for a while.

As soon as he reminded me what the doctors had said, I realized I had stumbled off the yellow brick road and I was never going back to Kansas, at least not for a very long time. He was right. No one had told me I could go back to work. No one had recommended it. But in my heart, getting a job felt like the right thing to do. Of course, it did. Getting a job always felt like the right thing for me to do. It gave me money, self-respect, satisfaction, and challenges. Until I had gotten sick, to a large degree, it had defined who I was. I wasn't just Linda Meilink or even Linda Valine[4], baby boomer, mother of three, college grad, and driver of an old Ford Escort down life's increasingly crowded highway. I was Linda Meilink, executive editor of the Paradise Post. Linda Meilink, writer. Linda Meilink, columnist. Linda Meilink, journalism teacher and mentor of a couple of dozen young journalists. Linda Meilink, charging lunch with the mayor on my company credit card. Linda Meilink, slightly older, blonde version of Lois Lane. Linda Meilink, features editor at the Reno Gazette-Journal. Linda Meilink, board member of the California Society of Newspaper Editors. When I got sick, I became Linda Meilink, nobody.

I had a doctor's appointment the day after my job interview, and Kevin insisted on going with me to hear what the doctor would think about my career plans. I smiled, cajoled, and pleaded. All right, in the end, I begged.

But Dr. Russell, the pain specialist, didn't budge. "We did discuss that, at some point, you might be able to return to work, but I don't see that happening for at least six months and then only part-time."

"I'm afraid you are just setting yourself up for failure," she continued. "How will you feel if you have to quit this job?"

"What if I just have a strong feeling in my heart that this is the right thing to do?"

She sighed. She respected that. Mentally, it would probably cheer me up and give me a boost of confidence, at least initially. But there

4   My legal name, which I assumed after my marriage

was no way I could keep it up past a few weeks. Actually, I wouldn't last a few days.

As I remember it, I was pretty quiet all the way home. Kevin didn't say, "I told you so." He didn't have to. I felt like he was being smug. I was angry at him, the doctor, and even the editor at the *Modesto Bee*. How crazy was that for her to try to hire a disabled woman?

I had to call and tell the *Bee* that I couldn't take the job, if it were offered. Luckily, when I called, I got an answering machine and told it that my doctor said I couldn't go back to work for quite a while and I would call back when I could go back to work. I knew I shouldn't have left a message. I should have waited until I had a live voice at the other end. There are rules about leaving messages. It's okay to call to confirm lunch or set up an appointment, but it's not okay to tell a potential employer that you can't take a job, especially after you sat for two hours convincing him or her that you were the best and the only qualified candidate for the job. I owed her a personal phone call, but I couldn't do it. I was too afraid I would cry. Once again, I found myself unable to say good-bye. I may have been stoic at times about the pain, but I was never stoic about the loss of my job.

We've Come a Long Way

Several hundred years ago in Italy, a popular pre-surgery anesthetic was to put a wooden bowl over the patient's head and beat on it until the patient passed out.

I called my sister Darlene and wept bitterly. "Why did this happen to me?"

Three years later, I have at least a partial answer. If I had been able to keep that job, could I have ever written this book? Would I be able, as I am now, to take the time each morning to steep in a hot bath to get my muscles circulating to make sure I can do the things I need to do to keep my mind and body healthy?

You are not your job. As I look around now at most employed professionals, I admire them, but I also think they are just a bit crazy. I no longer have to have the large paycheck or a staff of subordinates to prove I am somebody. Besides, my home office is even larger than the one I had at work.

As I write this, I am looking at the roses on my patio. I not only can stop to smell them, but I have time to tend them, keep them healthy, feed them, and snip some off for a homegrown bouquet. So if you have to give up your job, be patient. After a while, you can get used to it. And you won't have a crisis when you retire.

A lonely woman is a dog's best friend.

Susie Croley

Chapter Twelve

Pet Me

Staying at home and not working was lonely, although I admit that, at first, the loneliness was kind of lovely. There was no long list of phone calls waiting to be returned, no lengthy meetings, and no calendars with items scratched out and rewritten and then rewritten again. There was no Rotary Club, where I had to break bread with a few friends and a multitude of middle-aged men with traditional values who hated me and thought I should be at home cleaning the sink.

The first few months of being at home is like a hiatus. You keep expecting that you are going back somewhere and the time you have to reflect and relax is valuable. But as time goes by, you realize there really is nowhere to go, your co-workers stop calling to see how you are, and your friends are busy with demanding jobs of their own. Then you realize that your time isn't valuable at all. It's not time stolen from a busy life of responsibilities. It's cheap. It's free. It's like afternoon soap operas, which would be boring except there is so little else to excite you. It's as predictable as black heels with a black dress, as uncomfortable as old socks with a hole in the toe.

And friends and family who are struggling to balance work, home, and social lives look at you with envy, not with sympathy for the diabolic pain that plays like a loud, screeching background noise in your oth-

Getting the Right Pet for You

Check out the breed (or breeds) of the dog you are getting or talk to a dog trainer. Different breeds have different needs. Some need a great deal of exercise; others are couch potatoes. Some need plenty of grooming; others just need an occasional bath. If you are five feet tall and weigh ninety pounds, a Rottweiler may be a great guard dog, but, when leashed, he could knock you over if he sees an attractive female.

erwise uneventful days. Some of them are so stressed and so unaware of how bad you feel that there are days when they think they'd like to trade places with you.

And I wish they could, but, in the meantime, I needed a companion. I needed someone who would:

- Keep me company but not ask me any questions.
- Not want to go to the movies or out for coffee.
- Listen without judging.
- Look in my in the eyes on bad days with an expression that said, "I care. I understand."

In short, I needed a dog. At an online site where patients rate their own therapies and treatments, pet therapy was listed at one time as number two on a list of most effective therapies, at 9.2 out of 10, as of January 2007. The only remedy found to be more valuable than pet therapy was patient education from Web sites, rated at 9.5 out of 10.

The results of this unscientific online poll, with the most tried-and-true drugs like amitriptyline ranking a dismal 5.1 and even acupuncture rated no higher than 5.6, are probably more indicative of how poorly conventional and alternative remedies perform than they are about how well a pooch can solve your worst nightmares.

But once I begin to scout the Web sites where homeless dogs are listed like jilted lovers on Match.com, I could not be dissuaded. I had to have a dog. Kevin, who is much wiser than I am and tends to avoid impulsive, irresponsible, and reckless decisions, emphatically did not want a dog. He didn't want a little, yappy dog that would get under his feet and on his nerves. He didn't want a big, bone-crunching dog that would sail through windows and fill our backyard with giant turds.

He asked how I would take care of a dog. I could hardly get out of bed. Who would walk the dog, feed him, and take him to the vet? But in my pain-laden, drug-filled fantasy, our dog was going to sleep happily at my feet, except late at night when Kevin was at work. Then he would defend me from burglars, rapists, or the neighborhood teenagers who were throwing beer cans in my front yard.

In the end, Kevin indulged me. We went online and found the perfect dog. He was a handsome, shepherd-Rottweiler mix that was about two years old and currently in an animal rescue center. His keeper said he weighed about forty pounds.

Of course, his foster father was lying about the dog. He was huge, ninety pounds carved out of at least twenty-six various breeds, none smaller than an Alaskan husky. But he was being kept on a concrete slab in the one-hundred-degree sun. We looked at each other, and we looked at the cage. We couldn't leave him there. The next thing we knew, we were on our way home with the dog occupying the entire backseat of Kevin's Toyota, which terrified both of us. His body odor and bad breath filled the entire car.

Kevin named him Hambone. The first time we left him alone, he jumped through a screen and got out. The next time we went away, we closed the windows. In a desperate attempt to get out of the home we had so generously provided him, he ate the woodwork off three doors.

When we saw the narrow strips of wood and shredded plaster, we thought someone had used an ax to try to break down the door. It was that bad. It was a few minutes before we figured out what had happened. It gave new meaning to the phrase, "Grandma, what big teeth you have!"

As for Hambone, he was thrilled to see us. He wagged his tail as if to say, "Gosh, I'm so glad you're home. I was so worried I had to eat all the woodwork off the doors, and I still couldn't get out."

That wasn't the worst of it. He got diarrhea from eating the paint, and the paint in his stool ruined our new carpet. I called the woman who ran the dog rescue center, and her advice was to get another dog as a companion, which, she assured us, would quell his anxiety.

That's how we got Sadie. She was only sixty pounds, as friendly and self-assured as Hambone was anxious. It was an arranged marriage, but it worked out. Now we had two big dogs, and taking care of them was a huge problem. There were days when I had been too sick to walk them, and dogs need exercise. And, to put it delicately, they don't use the toilet. This means bending over or squatting down on knees and ankles that don't like to be disturbed. It means getting up with a sick dog in the night. It means driving them to the vet on days when you've taken the maximum amount of medications, and taking them to the vet means big money that could be used at a spa for a nice pedicure. It means your spouse, if you have one, will have to join in and help with chores he or she really did not want to do.

So before you jump in and get a pet to join you for tea each afternoon at 3:00, think carefully about what you are doing. I have known pet lovers who spent their last dime on expensive medication for their pet. Will you have to decide on who gets the meds, you or your pet? If you live alone, visualize what it will be like when your dog has a bout of diarrhea when you can hardly get out of bed.

I would love to give you a happy ending here, but, when Kevin began working long hours every day, I had a long flare, Hambone ate the woodwork again, Sadie became incontinent, and both of us developed severe allergies to the dog hair, we had to find homes for our dogs. We were heartbroken. You may prefer an outdoor cat as a better pet.

I have read articles in magazines in veterinarian's offices that assure readers that having a pet will allow you to live longer and stay in better mental health. And for those who must have pets, I wish them well. I really do. But pets are expensive. They are work. If you have time and energy, you might try what works for me. You could write a book instead.

Not everyone will be receptive or supportive.

Chronic Fatigue Syndrome and Fibromyalgia

Chapter Thirteen

My (Former) Best Friends

"When it hurts, how long does the pain last?" my friend asked as we sat at Starbucks sipping low-fat mochas.

"It hurts all the time."

"All the time? Like now? Does it hurt now?"

"Yes."

"Did it hurt while you were walking down the street?"

"Yes."

"When we were shopping, did it hurt then?"

"Yes. It hurts all the time."

"Well, you look fine."

Then a few weeks later, she said, "Why don't you come over here? I don't feel like driving."

"It hurts too much to drive."

"What do you mean? I thought you said you were cooking."

"I am cooking. But when I'm done, I'll be exhausted. And cooking isn't the same as driving. My leg hurts when I hold my foot on the gas."

"Why does that hurt?"

"I don't know. It just does."

That was a conversation with my best friend several years ago. Now we don't talk at all. She always said that, for someone who was sick, I looked fine. I guess I still look fine. She was my best friend for years, and I still miss her. She's a decade older than I am and still in vibrant health. I'm not sure she ever really believed in my illness. I certainly don't think she ever understood how intolerable the pain was.

She wasn't exactly one of those perpetually optimistic friends where everything is rosy. Frankly, before I got sick, that's what I liked about her. She was funny, sarcastic, and critical with a biting wit. Like me, she was a writer.

When I was healthy, I really enjoyed and appreciated her frankness. Like most writers, I had learned that honest feedback was rare. Most friends, co-workers, and family are more polite than honest when asked for an opinion. No, that dress doesn't make you look fat. Yes, I loved your most recent poem. Really, that rug in your living room doesn't clash with the painting on your wall.

She was never shy about offering her opinions. She had once told me I had no artistic taste whatsoever. I shrugged it off because I didn't think much of her preferences either. We disagreed on many things, and she was often abrasive, but I didn't take it personally ... until now. It was another thing about me that the disease had changed. Where I once wanted sparkling wit and acerbic commentary, now I needed a kind word and a soft shoulder. When I was the features editor in Reno, my friend had a lot to say about what I should be doing better. It hurt, especially because I felt so helpless. There were times she offered to make dinner for me, but I was always too tired to drive over after work for coffee, or conversation.

But I believe she thought I was avoiding her, inventing excuses for not following through with plans we'd made. Even though I apologized profusely, I am sure she felt rejected. And until you've experienced chronic pain, it's difficult for those in good health to contemplate what it is like. After all, I looked okay.

Like many others, she suggested ways that she thought I might overcome my disability. She told me a few times that she had learned how to turn off pain by meditating. I felt she thought I was overplaying my hand, looking for sympathy. If I just sat and thought about it, I could learn to put the pain in the back of my mind, like she had done. I'm sure I didn't appreciate it.

I was in pain, and she didn't understand. But the loss of that friendship was mostly my fault. I didn't know yet how to communicate very well about what was going on with me. I was moody and depressed. One day, I was desperate for attention. The next day, I wanted to be alone.

In the end, I was the one who blew up at her. Our birthdays are a week apart. I canceled, telling her that I didn't need anyone else to make me feel bad enough about myself. I felt bad enough already.

I was distraught. I needed friends more than ever, but I needed a caregiver, the kind of friend who gives you a back rub and a pep talk. I hadn't really appreciated those qualities in a friend before because I didn't need them.

I wanted to apologize, but Kevin felt the stress of our relationship was just adding to my misery.

"Let it go," he told me.

She wasn't the only close friend I lost. During my years as editor at the *Paradise Post*, I had a confidante who was single, as I was, and with whom I discussed the really important things: men, clothes, diets, Botox, men, housecleaning, travel, men, careers, and men. She was younger than I was and extremely attractive with beautiful almond-colored hair and eyes. We occasionally went out dancing, or as her boss used to put it, "trolling for men." We talked on the phone almost daily and incessantly. She was my confidante for nearly a decade. We shared heartbreak when men didn't call and exhilaration when we were promoted. However, she was a staunch

Are You Lonesome Tonight?

There are an unlimited number of ways to enjoy yourself with other people, even if you're not in the best of health. For some, you have to be able to commit to one night a week. If you never know how you will be feeling, there are more flexible ways to make friends:

Join a gym. If you can't do anything else, just hang out at the pool.

Volunteer. Some organizations, especially political parties, need people to perform simple tasks, like making telephone calls.

Join a church or meditation group.

Sing in a choir.

Play pool or ping-pong at a Parks and Recreation building.

Connect with a fibromyalgia support group.

Join a writing group and write your memoirs.

Take cooking classes.

Sign up for one-day excursions through your Parks and Recreation Department.

Take up bingo!

Join a book club. Most bookstores offer them.

Become a sports fan and attend local games.

Make friends on the Internet.

Work the polls on Election Day.

Volunteer to tutor adults and children who have problems reading.

Attend any twelve-step meeting (and you don't have to have an addiction to benefit from their program)

Republican with a dim view of entitlement programs. I know she felt strongly that many, if not most, disability claims were fraudulent.

I had no doubt such people existed. I'm sure they still exist. But even though I am a born-and-raised Democrat and our voting ballots were as different as our hair color, we rarely let a day or two go by without checking in by phone. We took each other to lunch on our birthdays, ordering shamefully calorie-ridden desserts like chocolate mousse cake with ice cream and chocolate sauce.

When I first started seeing a doctor and was told I had carpal tunnel and tendonitis, she was sympathetic. But when I went on sick leave for the first time, things got a little sticky. I could sense her disapproval. I felt just like another one of those whiners.

I sensed she thought, at the very least, that I was exaggerating my illness and learned to steer the conversations around it. Then I left for Florida. When I came back to California and got married, I assumed we would resume our friendship. That didn't happen. She seemed reluctant to return my calls. When we made lunch dates, she canceled them. However, she did offer to sing at my wedding, and that meant a lot to me. You see, we had spent years bemoaning our single state, reassuring each other that our princes were still out there somewhere. Her faith that I would someday meet mine had cheered me up many times. In one sense, I wanted to thank her for her support during all those years. I was even going to introduce her at the wedding and give a little speech about how much she had supported me in my search for the perfect man.

Then, two days before my wedding, as my sister and future husband and I were trying to decide on how to arrange the chairs to fit all the guests in the living room, she called to tell me she wasn't coming.

Over Fifty?

Here are some great ways to make new friends:

Move to an adult complex that offers classes and other activities.

Attend meditation classes.

Dress up and go dancing at senior centers. Even if you can't dance, there are always those who are sitting out who love to make conversation.

Check out your local seniors clubs.

Write your life story to pass down to your grandchildren!

Some universities allow seniors to attend classes without credit for a small fee. Not only will you make friends, you will be exercising your brain.

"I can't believe I'm doing this," she said by way of apology. Her new boyfriend and his son were going to a football game on Sunday, and they were invited to a tailgate party on Saturday. She told me her boyfriend's son would be terribly disappointed if she didn't go.

"Do you hate me?" she asked.

I guess I should have been gracious. I didn't yell at her, which might have been a better thing to do. I told her I would call her back and never did. She didn't send a present, and she's never called me.

It's hard for me to say whether my illness had something to do with the end of our friendship. Something changed after I got sick. Maybe it wasn't my illness. Maybe my marriage was the natural end of our friendship because we spent most of our time together trying to figure out how to get married. Because I don't talk to her anymore, I'll probably never know. I tried not to complain a lot about not feeling well, but maybe I did. Maybe it's just no fun to be around someone with chronic pain. I hate to think that, in the end, our relationship was that shallow, but maybe we no longer had the same thing in common, men and clothes. Or maybe I've just been a bitch since I've gotten sick. But I lost two very good friends.

Was I lonely? Yes, but only vaguely. If I had to trade a reduction in pain with the pleasure of company, I would have chosen the pain reduction. Most nights, I preferred resting with a good book. Even talking and listening were burdensome at times.

Still, I sometimes wish I hadn't given up on my friendships that easily. I think I should e-mail or call and say, "What happened?" Maybe someday I will.

Since then, I have improved and started making new friends. Of course, now I look for something more in a friend than sharp wit, a penchant for nice clothes, and a worry over wrinkles. One of the more fortunate side effects of the disease is that I learned that leaning on a friend could be just as comfortable as allowing friends to lean on you.

My sisters have been a constant source of comfort, especially because both of them have similar health problems. Not all family issues can be resolved, but, when I felt like I was ready to die, it occurred to me more than once that these people would cry at my funeral. There is probably no bond tighter than that. Do all my friends have fibromyalgia? Not at all. But everyone has something they need help with, and I'm glad there are still things I can do.

If you lose friends because of your illness, you're not really losing anything at all. Don't feel as if you have suddenly become undesirable to be around. Under these circumstances, don't take the loss of a friend personally.

If you can get out, participate in new activities like cooking classes and volunteering. You can also post listings on www.craigslist.com. I posted an ad looking for other fibromyalgia sufferers in my area, and that's how I met Sandra. Three to four percent of the population suffers from FMS, so you are bound to know someone who knows someone who is in the same physical and emotional state. When I talk to someone who has FMS, even a stranger, I have an instant bond that is deeper than any relationship I had with former tennis partners, occasional lunch mates, or co-workers.

Incidentally, you may find another annoying and subtle dynamic occurs if you are disabled. Friends, family, close friends, boyfriends, acquaintances, and near-to-perfect strangers will have no qualms about intruding on your time. They will ask you to watch Oprah for them and give them the skinny. They will ask you to meet them for lunch ten minutes from now. They will take up hours of your time droning on about work problems. After all, it isn't as if you are doing anything. When I mentioned this to Kevin, he said, "Oh God! I do the same thing to you myself. I always figure you aren't busy, and I interrupt you all the time."

His admission made me feel relieved because I sometimes felt put-upon while wanting a social life at the same time. I wanted to feel useful. But like everyone else, I was tired of being called at the last minute, as if my friend's lunch date had fallen through, but I could always be relied on to be there.

When I tell friends and family I am busy, they often ask, "Doing what?" Hardly anyone ever asked me that while I was working.

Many times, I have been so frustrated because I have been lonely for days and someone calls just as I am leaving for the doctor's office to ask me for coffee. I will say, "Well, let's set a time and date for another day," but they usually decline. They are "pretty busy" right now and will call "when they have some free time."

If you know how to handle this problem, please send me an email (lindameilink@aol.com) and let me know how you solved it. I haven't a clue. And if I don't get back to you right away, it's because I am busy.

The divorce rate for a chronically ill person is an astounding 75 percent.

*Chronic Fatigue Syndrome, Fibromyalgia
and Other Invisible Illnesses*

Chapter Fourteen

In Sickness and In Health

During the bleak days of my illness, I flew back to Toledo, Ohio, my hometown, to visit my sisters and brothers. My return flight arrived in Reno at 11:00 PM on Monday night. Flying can be excruciating for FMS patients. I'm not sure if it's sitting still, the nearly imperceptible vibration of the plane, or the bad air. Maybe it's a combination of all three. That night after I stumbled sleepily out of my tiny mid-row seat and down to the baggage claim, Kevin wasn't there to meet me. I was disappointed. He isn't always prompt, but I had hoped his anticipation of seeing me would have motivated him to get there before my plane came in.

My luggage came, but Kevin didn't. For an hour or so, I paced back and forth, rolling my suitcase from the baggage check out to the sidewalk where cars were waiting, searching for him. I thought he had maybe mistaken the time.

Helpful Hint

There's probably no better time to get marriage counseling than when your spouse is also your caregiver.

I began to worry. His mother had died in her sleep of a heart attack when she was forty-eight. Kevin was sometimes late, but never this late. He wasn't the kind of husband who would forget to pick me up. I thought about calling him, but my cell phone was dead. I dragged my suitcase back into the airport, but I couldn't find a phone, and it hurt too much to search for one. I couldn't walk that far.

I finally hailed a cab. By now, I was afraid to go home. I was sure he had died. I mentally prepared myself for the worst. What would I do if he were unconscious or worse? But when we pulled up in front of my house, the lights and the television set were on. Kevin opened the door. Dirty shirts and socks, piles of books, old magazines, and newspapers were strewn everywhere. The house looked just like it did in his bachelor days. He also needed a shave and a shower.

"Why didn't you pick me up?" I asked.

"You told me your plane came in Tuesday," he said. It was Monday.

"Why would I do that?" I had too much adrenalin pumping to have a rational conversation. "You forgot to pick me up! How could you?"

"Before you left, you told me Monday," he said. "But when I asked you over the weekend, you said Tuesday."

"Well, if you were confused, why didn't you call me?"

"Because you said you were coming in Tuesday."

I don't remember what else I said before I pulled on my pajamas and got out of bed. When he came in the bedroom and started to undress, I told him I didn't want him to sleep with me. I was still too angry and mentally distraught to have him lie next to me, listening to his even breathing while I was still fuming.

"You'll have to sleep in the other room," I said.

He picked up his pillow and got out. I lay there alone, remembering the terror I had felt when I thought he had died. After a half hour or more, I couldn't stand it. I wanted him to be there to reassure myself he was still with me. I went back to the spare room where Kevin was sleeping.

"I'm sorry," I said without apologizing, my voice just slightly more civil. "I can't sleep without you in my bed. You're going to have to get up and get back in bed with me."

I didn't think he would, but he very dutifully got in bed, picked up his pillow, and padded down the hall in his bare feet. When he got into bed and put his arms around me, I started to cry.

"I thought you were dead," I said, sobbing.

My world was confusing, even terrifying. I realized for the first time that one word, misspoken, could cause a dog to charge the mailman or a surgeon to botch an operation. The wrong word has more repercussions than I could ever have imagined. And I lived in a world where wrong words kept dropping in and I didn't notice. I didn't even hear them until it was too late.

You would think I would have immediately recognized the fibromyalgia syndrome. I knew that I often substituted one word for another. I had done this for years. But I needed to believe his forgetfulness was all his fault. I was also angry because he seemed so satisfied without me when I came home unexpectedly. It fanned my worse fear, that he secretly wanted to get rid of me, I was useless to him, and the only thing that tied him to me was his sense of guilt.

I don't know anyone with FMS who hasn't felt this way. Even though I try hard to do my share of housework, errands, and gainful employment, what I can contribute is often much less than half.

And I am fortunate. I still manage to get some of the housework done, and Kevin is happy to take over when I can't. He does the heavy grocery shopping and pays the bills because I am prone to forget.

He has learned to accommodate my illness. I sometimes still have what we call spells, where I become disoriented and extremely forgetful. I can feel them coming on most of the time.

You Can Be Invaluable!

No matter what else you do, you can become what every spouse secretly wants most ... a good listener!

Now that my pain is greatly reduced most days, I seem to be more aware of them. They come and go like a migraine, and I suspect some neurological damage may be causing them. I try to let him know what is going on before we get in an argument, before I get lost on the freeway, or throw a temper tantrum because I can't find my keys. When he finds the checkbook in a bathroom drawer or my glasses on the top shelf of the bookcase, he doesn't criticize me anymore.

But, despite his thoughtfulness and consideration, I resent him sometimes. I watch him go to work each day in a career that I loved. There was a time when I could have bought whatever I wanted without consulting him. Now I feel like I am asking his permission because he is the primary breadwinner.

I know there are days when he wishes he could stay home all day like I do, sitting around in his pajamas. He sometimes works overtime because we need the money. I hate the fact that I don't pay my own way. I realize he pays for the food I eat. I feel dependent and try to feel grateful, but that's not what my idea of marriage should be. It should be a contract between two equal partners.

Even though we have insurance, my illness is expensive. There are acupuncture treatments and massages that aren't covered, co-payments for drugs and doctor's visits, and over-the-counter medications.

As time goes on, I've become more comfortable with the inequalities, but it doesn't stop me from feeling insecure. Kevin is the world's nicest guy. And he is loyal. Knowing that he wouldn't leave me because of my illness is reassuring, but it also raises questions. Would he leave if I were well? How can I ever be sure that he is happy?

The first year we were together, Kevin had physical problems of his own, and he has often said he didn't think we would be together if we hadn't gotten sick. He teases me and says he was too sick to chase me and I was too sick to run away. This doesn't sound very good as a foundation for a happy marriage. Nevertheless, it is probably true. He was a bachelor at forty-four, and I had been divorced and single for twenty years. We were an unlikely match, both commitment-phobic, extremely independent, stubborn, and in need of a lot of downtime. We like to be alone a lot. Our fantasy is to live in a duplex someday, one of us in each unit.

Even my illness inspired his proposal. One afternoon as I cooked dinner, he leaned against the counter, watching me. We were talking about the high cost of health insurance when he said casually, "I guess we should get married. I mean, it just makes sense. That way I can put you on my health insurance at work."

"Are you proposing?" I asked as I finished stirring the mushrooms and onions and opened the oven to check on the chicken.

"Well," he said awkwardly with his arms folded. He was leaning so far back into the counter that he almost knocked over the blender. "I guess I am."

Fibromyalgia upstaged me at my wedding. I had two women, friends on my husband's side, who followed me around all day, wanting to discuss my symptoms because they thought they might have FMS. It was awkward, and I had to keep excusing myself to spend time with other guests, who all wanted to know how I was holding up. It seemed everyone was more interested in my illness than in me.

Stressed Spouses?

Sure, you're suffering, but having a spouse who is ill can be devastating. The Well Spouse Foundation offers support at www.wellspouse.org.

And it ruined my wedding night. We were married in our home. By the time the guests left, I was flat on the bed, too tired to move and so sore that Kevin couldn't put his arm around me.

And I am lucky. Many FMS patients have spouses who don't believe in their illness or think they exaggerate. I recently had a conversation with a woman who left her husband because he insisted she wasn't really disabled and wanted her to continue working and keeping house for him. It happens all the time.

There are spouses who get tired of listening to complaints or simply don't like the company of anyone who is less than able because it's depressing. You can't go on that ski trip or even stay up all night watching bad movies.

Kevin often has asked me to do something simple, like accompany him while he walks the dogs, but I wasn't even able to do that. We used to bicycle together, take trips to the beach, and kayak. When I am in remission, we can do those things again. But it's been a long haul.

Some people like to be taken care of. Some doctors and health practitioners have told me that's one factor that keeps FMS patients from recovering. They don't want to give up being a patient. I find it hard to believe. Would a doctor ever remark that a patient with a broken leg was preventing his leg from healing? I guess the hypothetical broken-leg patient could be reluctant to get up and walk around and participate in therapy, but I don't think he or she could stop the leg from healing.

In any event, I don't really care for being a patient, and I am a very bad one. At my very worst, I look for someone else to blame and refuse to listen to reason, just like I did that night in Reno when Kevin didn't show up at the airport after I told him to come on the wrong day.

Most women with fibromyalgia get divorced. I don't know what the statistics are on men. But my husband married me during the worst days of my illness. I've known other women with FMS who have found true love after they were diagnosed. So if you are single, don't think that no one will want you.

If you have a husband who is kind and considerate, appreciate him, even if he always loses the cap for the toothpaste and hogs the covers.

Again, which came first, fibromyalgia or depression? That question continues to puzzle many researchers, who have found that the two illnesses have similar characteristics. Many people with fibromyalgia are depressed. Conversely, depressed people often complain of unexplainable aches and pains along with fatigue and an inability to stay asleep at night. At some point researchers find depression present in the majority of fibromyalgia patients. In fact, more than 25 percent of patients do have depression when fibromyalgia is diagnosed.

Harris H. McIlwain, MD,
and Debra Fulghum Bruce,
The Fibromyalgia Handbook:
A 7-Step Treatment to Halt
and Even Reverse Fibromyalgia

Chapter Fifteen

Paging Dr. Kevorkian

After I quit my job in Reno, Kevin left to take a better job in Modesto. It was a bad time for a move, but a great time for a better job because only one of us was working. He was gone for the whole month of January. He came home on weekends, but I needed him every day. If there was ever a time I shouldn't have been alone, it was then.

The pain swelled like a boil about to burst. Pretty soon, it encompassed everything. I stayed in bed, trying unsuccessfully to read and sometimes trying to meditate. I used ice bags and hot packs. I walked the floor. I added over-the-counter drugs like Alka-Seltzer, thinking some combination of drugs might at least lessen the pain. I was obsessed, or perhaps I should say possessed, by the pain. I was no longer really in my right mind. I would open a can of soup, put it on the stove, and forget it until I smelled it burning. I don't even remember what I ate for that whole month, although I think I put away a lot of ice cream.

The pain was the first thing I felt in the morning and the last thing I felt at night. I would try to put it in the back of my mind so I could get to sleep. It was with me whenever I took a step, turned my head, and bent down to pick up the morning newspaper. I never had a moment when I could relax, take a deep breath, and stretch out without the pain. It was more constant than an unrelenting toothache, sharper than a bad cut. It interrupted

To Sleep, Perchance To Dream?

Hamlet may have been mad, but even he knew there was something sinister about suicide. If you've ever thought that an overdose was a nice peaceful way to die, think again. Most of the time, an overdose triggers vomiting. You end up choking to death on your vomit. By comparison, a day of chronic pain isn't so horrible after all.

my thinking, sleeping, phone conversations, exercise, plans, and best intentions.

When Kevin called, I tried not to alarm him. Fortunately, he was doing well at his new job. I counted days until he came home, but, when he came home for a weekend, the pain didn't diminish. I didn't even find solace in his company. Nothing. The pain had swallowed my whole life. I tried to think of something I might want to do before I died, and the only thing I could think of was seeing my grandkids. Yeah, I thought bitterly, like I would have the strength to travel. And there were days when even that didn't matter.

Pretty soon, I began plotting my own suicide. I had no great passion for dying. I didn't feel like Madame Butterfly or even Madame Bovary. There were no grand soliloquies, "to be or not to be," fantasies about heaven, consolation of one hundred virgins or even getting to be one of them, or fear of hell. In fact, I wanted to get out of hell. I was not excited or fearful. Maybe I would wake up somewhere else, but, hey, if I didn't, that would be okay, too.

There was, however, the small problem of the grief of my husband, my sisters and brothers, my children, and the sadness of my grandchildren growing up without remembering their grandmother. I had lost both my grandfathers before I was born, and it left a hole in my life somehow. It was a small hole, but a painful one nevertheless.

And my family and friends would all feel guilty. "If only I had called her that day," they would think. "I didn't know she was that sick," they would tell each other, their cold hands holding those little cards that say "In Memory Of ..." as they sat at the funeral home. They would say, "I wish she had told me."

But that was irrelevant. No sympathetic phone call, not even several of them, could fix the problem. As it was, my sisters Darlene and Suzie listened to me sob after I lost my job. And they were wonderful to me. So this made me feel guiltier because I knew how much they would be hurt if they knew I was thinking of killing myself and causing them so much grief.

There was only one way out. It had to look like an accident. For the first time, I understood why some drivers lose control of the car while doing eighty on the freeway and crash into an abutment. I didn't drive much then, but, on the days that I drove to see Maureen, I began to look for places where I could crash without a chance of survival. Surviving as an invalid would make it worse, if that were possible. I sometimes thought about driving up in the mountains and missing one of the quirky turns alongside a nearly endless drop-off. It would be kind of like *Thelma and Louise*, but without the romantic underpinnings. There was nothing romantic about this.

I am certainly not a mystic, but it seemed I could sense the presence of my mother and father, who are both deceased. I dreamed about them often, and I could sense their disapproval. My mother had suffered with chronic pain for decades before she died. My father died, gasping for breath, of emphysema. I

More Work, More Pain?

The National Center for Health Statistics reports that between 1996 and 2006, there was a 38 percent increase in workers throughout the United States who suffered chronic pain.

also dreamed about a childhood friend of mine who had died recently, who kept trying to tell me it wasn't my time yet. If you are a skeptic, you might say my perceived presence of my parents was a manifestation of my own subconscious guilt. You know, since I've been sick, these kind of debates don't interest me. I don't know whether there is a supernatural, subconscious, or collective consciousness. These feelings were there, whatever they were, and they did make me hesitate – at least a bit.

The only person I told about my suicidal plans was Maureen, and she was alarmed, although she tried not to show it. I was calm when I explained all this to her. I had lived a good life so far. I had three wonderful, successful kids. I had had a great career. I wasn't afraid anymore. After all, we all have to check out sometime. Why not check out when you have nothing in particular to fear anymore? When you have nothing to live for?

My dispassionate response to her alarm frustrated her. "What if this is part of your karma and you find you have to come back and do this all again?"

I had never seen her angry before. "What if there is no karma?" I asked. "What if you die and you're just dead, and it doesn't hurt anymore?"

"Is that what you think happens? And what if you're wrong?"

After she put the needles in and left me for my twenty-minute treatment, she told me to think about a time in my life when I was peaceful and happy and to go back there. I thought about lying on a sailboat in the San Francisco Bay. I thought about holding my children in my arms for the first time. I thought about Kevin on our wedding day. It was only a glimpse, but what if one of those times were still out there in some indeterminate future? What if there was a treatment, if not a cure, for fibromyalgia someday? And what about sparing my husband and children a sudden and incomprehensible grief?

The acupuncture alleviated the pain a little, even though it never worked for very long any more. I had a few hours, at most, of slight relief. The pain returned as I drove home, but I didn't even notice the abutment that day. I felt too much like a guilty child.

I decided to wait until I was settled in my new home in Modesto with Kevin, until I had seen my children and grandchildren again. My pain doctor once told me that, when the pain became unbearable, I could just take a sleeping pill and knock myself out for a few hours. I decided to do that in lieu of suicide, and it has gotten me through my worst days.

Just one other note: I was always careful with my medicine. If I killed myself, it would be intentional, not an accident. At no time did I take a handful of pills and leave it to fate.

But my distress had given me something to consider. As I mentioned earlier, two of Dr. Kevorkian's patients had fibromyalgia. I didn't even know what FMS was when he helped them take their lives, but I remember thinking at the time, "That's stupid. What if they come up with a cure for it next year?"

Others have said, "Why did they kill themselves? It wasn't a fatal illness." Well, I guess that's why they did it.

But while I defend the right of someone in unbearable, hopeless suffering to end their own life, I think most of these deaths are preventable and often occur because their pain is undertreated. Doctors do have numerous options when it comes to treating chronic pain. I did improve. Even though I am not completely well, I realize a complete recovery may be within reach someday. And on good days, when I go for a long bicycle ride, lie on the swing in the backyard in the spring, or talk to my grandchildren, I am glad I waited.

But chronic pain can be a killer. I would not have considered suicide if I had known for certain that the pain was temporary and would eventually be alleviated. I didn't know that then because I had waited for too many years before consulting a pain specialist. I wasted too many years trying to push myself through the same routine I had when I was well. I refused to adapt. I had heard too many phrases like "conquer your pain" and "feel better fast."

As N. Gregory Hamilton, a practicing psychiatrist and co-founder of the Oregon-based Physicians for Compassionate Care, wrote in *The Truth about Chronic Pain*:

> Dr. Kevorkian is in jail, and that is where he needs to be ... basically, we can treat pain. We have had national expert after national expert come out to conferences here in Oregon and talk to the doctors, nurses and hospice workers about pain control. These experts basically say that pain is treatable, and that people do not need to die in unrelieved agony. Depression is treatable, and opiod analgesics, surgical and radiation procedures, anti-inflammatory and antispasmodic medicines are all very effective pain control. When we systematically treat people's fear and pain both, people do not need to be frightened into suicide.

Right or wrong, Kevorkian is no longer in jail. But what Dr. Gregory wrote is true:

Somehow, without ever giving up the belief that someday you will be completely recovered, you have to begin to recognize your pain as a part of your life and make accommodations for it. The nature of pain, as part of the body's alarm system, is that it will not allow itself to be pushed aside.

As it stands, most of us will have to make compromises. The willingness to compromise with your pain can be a huge factor in your recovery. Dr. Robert Jarvik, a pioneer in artificial heart technology, also addressed this in *The Truth about Chronic Pain*. "Nobody wants a mere modest improvement." And for most of us with fibromyalgia, adequate pain control, exercise, and self-care will lead to more than a modest improvement. He said he hopes chronic pain patients will find examples of others who have:

> [F]ocused and gotten good treatment for their pain, gotten the right result, come out on the other side,

had a life after the debilitating phase of chronic pain, started at ground zero and reached a livable place. That's something that can really help …

A person has to walk away from the pain-free past they've lost, not mourn the past, not complain. Once something has happened to them that's bad enough to give them chronic pain, they have to change their attitude. They have to take the best of what's left in their life, push the pain out, and don't complain about it.

I don't completely agree with the doctor. It's sometimes good to have someone to vent or complain to. And certainly all of us will grieve over what we have lost, whether those things are temporary or permanent.

But you do have to take the best of what's left in your life and learn to use your capabilities creatively. Only when I understood my limitations did my life start to meld together again. On a bad day, I can take it for what it is. I sometimes just cancel my engagements, if I have any, plump up my pillows, and take enough pain medication to relax, read a good book, or watch a movie. Now that's something most people in perfect health don't have the option of doing.

Dr. Rhoades admits the issue of doctor-assisted suicide is a complicated one. "I would never assist in a suicide. I can see personally why some people would rather be dead, but it's not my job to take life. The first rule of medicine is, 'First, do no harm.'"

Dr. Rhoades also pointed out that, every day, better medications are being developed. Every day, it looks more likely that fibromyalgia sufferers in the near future will lead more comfortable lives. "I believe fibromyalgia is caused by trauma. We treat several women for severe pelvic pain, and virtually every one of them has been raped. It's not that it's all in the head. The nervous system is like a stereo system, and it's like someone has turned up the amps. Instead of getting a normal response to any type of stimulus, you get pain."

He adds that FMS sometimes burns itself out, and some patients recover spontaneously. If a FMS patient ends it all, we will never know if he or she might have recovered.

Narcotic prescription pain medicines are not recommended for regular use in the treatment of fibromyalgia pain, since narcotics can be habit-forming, and it is likely that there will be a need to find a better long-term solution for pain control.

Harris H. McLain, MD,
and Debra Fulghum Bruce,
The Fibromyalgia Handbook:
A 7-Step Program to Halt
and Even Reverse Fibromyalgia

Chapter Sixteen

The Doctor Who Prescribed Motrin

We moved a few times since I've been ill. Our last move was Reno to Modesto. I advise someone with fibromyalgia who has found a decent doctor not to move anywhere. Sure, it was hard struggling with boxes I couldn't remember packing. Trying to find my way around a new town wasn't easy, especially when I often got lost just a few blocks from home. But nothing was as onerous as trying to find a new medical team.

We now had an HMO, although our insurance insisted on calling it "HMO-like." My primary care physician had to approve every specialist I saw. I was given a list and told to choose my primary care physician from it. We knew nothing about medical care in Modesto. A few of my husband's co-workers made suggestions. If you've ever been to a doctor or dentist that a friend referred, you will probably agree that it's amazing how personal and idiosyncratic our choices of personal care can be. One friend prefers a doctor because she's a woman; another prefers a doctor because he or she has a great bedside manner. Some even like doctors who share their interests; for example, golfing, tennis, or traveling. Some like doctors who dispense samples. I don't know. It just seems to me that picking a doctor is as personal as choosing a best friend. The last doctor I consulted based on a friend's advice got very angry when I asked her questions and advised me not to consult the Internet or other texts for that matter.

"If you don't trust what I'm telling you, why are you paying me?" she asked.

Why indeed? That was the last time I paid her.

The doctor I chose at random was young, svelte, and good-looking. He didn't have much to say to me, except I was taking too many drugs. His theory was that, if I went off the heavy stuff, Motrin and a glass of water would eventually do the trick. I guess I failed to convey how serious my pain was. His best advice for me was "mild aerobic exercise." I told him I did what I could, but he seemed to doubt it. Kevin, who came with me on the visit, asked him what he knew about fibromyalgia.

"Very little," he said.

I appreciated his honesty, but not his advice. I was tired of dealing with doctors who knew less about the disease than I did. I asked for referrals to a rheumatologist and a pain specialist. Rheumatologists generally treat anti-immune diseases like arthritis and lupus, but they are more likely than other specialists to know something about fibromyalgia. As of this writing, fibromyalgia doesn't fall under any specialty.

There were other problems getting medical attention as well. I could only be referred to specialists who were on our insurance plan. Once a specialist was found, I had to wait until the insurance approved the visit. Then, of course, there is generally a long wait for new patients, so it was a few months before I saw the rheumatologist. And what did she know about fibromyalgia?

"Nothing," she said.

She sometimes diagnosed it, but she didn't treat it. She treated arthritis. She couldn't treat it because she didn't really understand it. So she diagnosed me. She felt for sore spots, asked me questions, and then said, "You have classic fibromyalgia."

"I once prescribed steroids for a patient who had fibromyalgia, and she got better," she said hopefully. "Do you want to try steroids?"

I dutifully took my steroids for a few days, but, if anything, I felt worse. It was another dead end. In the meantime, I reapplied for disability insurance, another humiliating conversation about my inability to work. This time, I didn't cry.

My new family doctor also had trouble finding a pain doctor for me. Only a couple of pain specialists in our area accepted our insurance. I was finally referred to a neurologist in Stockton, about forty minutes away. A young doctor with a dispassionate expression told me he was a neurologist, not an anesthesiologist, and he refused to prescribe pain medication for me.

"I can't treat fibromyalgia because I don't know what it is," he said. "Light aerobic exercise and Motrin. Those are the only things I can prescribe for fibromyalgia."

I was beginning to wonder if there was a doctor in the region who was willing to treat me. I do understand the dilemma, of course. How does a doctor treat a condition he or she doesn't understand? But every day, doctors treat hundreds of other conditions, like Parkinson's or Alzheimer's disease, ALS, cancer, and so forth, disabling afflictions with no discernible cause or cure. So why not fibromyalgia?

To these doctors who suggested long walks and over-the-counter pain medicine, I explained I did light aerobic exercise when I could bear it, and Motrin had already been tried many times in the last eight years, with little or no effect.

When I explained to the neurologist that no one seemed to want to treat me, he asked, "So you have some aches and pains that come and go?"

Your Doctors' Records

It's extremely important that you see your physicians on a regular basis. If you must file for disability, social workers will ask for your records to help them determine the seriousness of your illness. Whether or not you are awarded SSI benefits depends to some degree on your doctor. If he or she sees fibromyalgia as little aches and pains, it is likely he or she will report that you are still able to work, no matter how ill you are. Make sure you have a doctor who understands your illness.

Well, not exactly. They never come because they never go away. And as for OTC medications, as Dr. Alina Garcia, fibromyalgia specialist, said, anyone whose pain can be controlled with Motrin probably doesn't have fibromyalgia. FMS pain is more like searing, hot, burning pain that comes and goes from one part of my body to another. And it never goes away. When I explained this to him, he seemed perplexed. I had the feeling that what I was telling him did not correspond to his concept of fibromyalgia. In his mind, he seemed to think it was a mild disorder that needed no special treatment.

I think he eventually believed me, especially when my husband chimed in to reinforce what I was saying. He nodded, thought about it for a minute, and then recommended a brain scan.

"You might have MS," he told me.

I left his office frightened and confused. I didn't know anything about MS, except that it sounded like an even more deadly than fibromyalgia.

"You don't have the classic symptoms of MS," he said, "but I think it is something you need to check."

As I pored over medical books and articles online, it was clear I didn't have classic symptoms of MS. In fact, I had only one symptom in common with MS sufferers, pain. MS is characterized by tremors, weakness, loss of sensation or numbness, blurred vision, and difficulty with balance, walking, and speaking.

In the absence of a clear diagnosis, doctors diagnose according to what they know. A neurologist believes you have MS or some other brain disorder. A chiropractor believes one of your vertebrae is out of place. A nutritionist believes you have a vitamin deficiency. A rheumatologist will tell you fibromyalgia is one of a group of disorders that include lupus, Lyme disease, and so forth. Somewhere I am sure there is a dentist who believes the problem can be fixed by cleaning your teeth.

Although the neurologist recommended a sleep study and brain scan, I elected not to have them. I was sure that both of them would lead to another dead end. Kevin objected, but not strenuously because he knew I was feeling pretty hopeless.

What I wanted and desperately needed was a doctor who would prescribe pain medication. Even though I was taking my medications at very low doses, I was running out. I could barely stand the pain now. What would happen if I couldn't find a doctor with any compassion or understanding of my condition?

This time, I called the only other local pain specialist covered under our insurance. I wanted to check him out before I went through the hassle of getting a referral, making an appointment, and driving to see him.

"Does this doctor treat fibromyalgia?" I asked the nurse.

"No," she said.

He'd never treated a fibromyalgia patient before. That seemed impossible to me. Everyone knows someone who has fibromyalgia. How could a pain doctor have no experience with them?

Actually, she told me, until very recently, this physician had only treated workers comp patients, and he had started a private practice.

She was sympathetic. Her mother had fibromyalgia. I asked if she would recommend this doctor for her mother.

"No," she said bluntly. "My mother sees a doctor in San Francisco."

In the meantime, I was still seeing the GP who was willing to prescribe Ambien, a sleeping pill, and Cymbalta, the antidepressant, but little else to deal with the pain. He said he did not prescribe controlled drugs. Despite the horrors of Cymbalta withdrawal, he believed it was a wonderful drug while Vicodin or Percocet were deadly drugs leading to addiction.

"Maybe you just need more exercise," he said one day as Kevin and I sat on stools at opposite ends of the tiny examining room.

"I do what I can," I told him with an edge in my voice.

"What you aren't seeing here," Kevin said, "is how severe the pain is. There are days when I have to help her get out of bed. She sometimes reaches down and grabs her leg with her hands to lift it so she can get out of the car."

"Hmm," he said. And he nodded.

Doctors take men more seriously. When I tried to tell this doctor how badly I hurt, I fell into the category of neurotic, menopausal female, but, when Kevin agreed with me, then maybe I wasn't so crazy after all. Still, he didn't seem to have any other solutions. He repeated that some patients seemed to do well on Motrin.

The intensity of fibromyalgia pain varies from one patient to another, but many doctors don't realize that. If Dr. White sees Mrs. Smith, who describes her pain as "little aches and pains," and then sees Mrs. Jones, who says she is ready to die rather to continue suffering, Dr. White will give Mrs. Smith a little Valium and tell her to try Motrin. Then he will give Mrs. Jones the same, along with "the positive thinking, learn-to-live-with-it, quit complaining, and so forth" speech.

Three months had gone by. I had seen three approved doctors in our HMO, and none of them would even give me a refill for my pain medicine. I was almost out of pain meds, and I was feeling pretty frantic so I even thought about driving back to Reno to see my pain specialist. I would have to pay for it and the pain medication out of my own pocket. And I would have to stay overnight because it was too far for me to drive there and back the same day. Still, I didn't have much choice, so I called and made an appointment.

The more I thought about the situation, the angrier I became. It was our insurance company's responsibility to provide me with medical care for my fibromyalgia, and not one of the doctors I had seen knew how to treat it. They had all openly admitted it.

I decided to fight back. I called my insurance company, explained the situation, and told them that I planned to file a grievance. It had been four months since I had seen a doctor who was competent in treating fibromyalgia. I had been without a physician's care all that time. I told them I wanted to go to a pain clinic listed in the Yellow Pages where the doctor advertised that he treated fibromyalgia. This was Central Valley Pain Clinic, which Dr. Rhoades ran. To my surprise, without an argument, the insurance rep authorized my visits.

Of course, I had to return to my primary care physician to get the referral. Then the problem was getting the appointment. It was May. The earliest appointment they had was August. I accepted it gratefully. I was fortunate enough to get an appointment at the pain clinic. But I was due to run out of medicine before my appointment. I went back to my family practitioner.

"Here's the problem," I said. "I am out of Vicodin. I have lots of other drugs like Percocet and Ultram. I don't like to take them because they make me feel woozy and drunk, but, if you don't refill my prescription for Vicodin, I'm going to have to take them because I don't have enough Vicodin to last until August."

He refilled my prescription. "But this is the last time." He handed me the slip of paper and walked out of the office.

Sure, I felt like a drug addict, but I was past caring. No one knew what kind of pain I had, certainly none of my doctors. For chronic pain, no other specialist can substitute for a competent pain specialist who sees patients like you every day and understands your chemistry. A pain doctor is probably the most essential specialist on your medical team.

Dr. Rhoades says it's pretty common for physicians who don't know what to do with a patient to send him or her somewhere else to get him or her out of his or her hair. If doctors don't want to treat chronic pain, they should refer them out.

There are two main reasons why patients are undermedicated:

- The doctors are afraid of losing their licenses or going to jail if they unwittingly become involved in some illegal drug activity.
- They are afraid the patients will become addicts.

There have been cases where physicians have ended up in jail or had their licenses pulled. Most states monitor doctors prescribing patterns. If you prescribe controlled substances, you have to take certain precautions and keep impeccable records. Not all physicians are willing to do that.

You need to find a doctor who cares more about your comfort and well-being than anything else. Isn't that what doctors are supposed to do?

Upon evaluation, your doctor will want to have a few basic laboratory tests taken to be sure no other serious medical problems are present. But these tests are limited in number and can be performed at your doctor's office or your local laboratory. They can usually be done at one visit.

Harris H. McIlwain, MD,
and Debra Fulghum Bruce,
*The Fibromyalgia Handbook:
A 7-Step Program to Halt
and Even Reverse Fibromyalgia*

Chapter Seventeen

What Would You Give for a Good Night's Sleep?

Just when I felt things could not get any worse, after I had lost my job and moved to Modesto only to find that giving up the stress of my job had only moderately improved my symptoms, Lowell, who had been following my progress, or lack thereof, gave me a call. He felt I needed better medical care, the best. He wanted me to go to a teaching hospital, like the University of California at Davis, for a consultation.

"What's the best medical treatment for fibromyalgia?" he asked.

I wasn't sure.

"Find the best place," he said, "and I will pay for your consultation."

I wasn't sure what to say. Part of me, embarrassed I couldn't afford such expensive treatment myself, wanted to say, "No, that's okay." By now, I was so discouraged that I didn't think anything would help anyway. Hadn't I read every self-help book on the market and consulted over a dozen doctors?

For a split second, I thought about declining. I didn't want to waste his money. Maybe part of me was afraid to try again and be disappointed once more. But I couldn't think of a logical reason to decline. And I sensed he wouldn't be pleased if I did. He isn't the type to make grand gestures. He wants results. Overwhelmed, I stammered out an acceptance.

When I hung up, I cried. He had told me once that having money was better than being poor, not so much because you could indulge yourself, but because it gave you more options. This type of medical care was an option I had not even considered. I had grown up and lived my adult life in a system where you took whatever medical care was

165

available to you. Sure, I had wanted the best, but, in the end, I would have been happy with a doctor who understood my illness, sympathized with my distress, and was willing to refill my pain medication.

Lowell's offer gave me hope, hope I didn't even realize I had lost. In the last six months, I had tried to lower my expectations. I began to accept the fact that I would never work full-time again. I would never be pain-free. I would probably never wake up feeling refreshed from a good night's sleep. Surely there were doctors somewhere that might be able to help. But where would I find them?

I decided to e-mail Kristin Thorson, the publisher of *Fibromyalgia Network*. In her quarterly publication, her writers interpret the most recent research papers published in medical journals and keep in touch with the latest research centers. Did she know where I could find the best fibromyalgia treatment?

"Stanford Medical Center Sleep Disorders Clinic," she replied.

I was surprised and not all that confident in her recommendation. Research specialists had often hinted at a link between fibromyalgia and sleep disorders, and I had read of some doctors who had achieved some degree of success in treating fibromyalgia patients who had underlying sleep problems. There were several studies, but, as far as I knew, nothing conclusive. I was already being treated for a sleep disorder. Wasn't I taking sleeping pills? I had tried several drugs for sleep, but none of them improved my symptoms. I was very skeptical. Shouldn't I go somewhere that took more of a general overview of the disease rather than limiting the treatment to a sleep disorder?

I had no idea that, as fibromyalgia specialist Paul Brown points out in his foreword to *Alternative Treatments for Fibromyalgia & Chronic Fatigue Syndrome* by Mari Skelly and Andre Helm, "The possible presence of thyroid disease, growth hormone deficiency, sleep apnea, other medical conditions, and some medications, which can all cause sleep apnea, shouldn't be overlooked. In one study, eleven of the forty-six women diagnosed with FM had another disorder that actually caused their pain."

I was extremely naïve. I didn't believe I had sleep apnea any more than I believed I had flat feet. I thought I knew my own body. I never woke up short of breath. Well, it was only a few times, and then I thought I was claustrophobic or having a bad dream.

And even though I knew a great deal about fibromyalgia, I didn't know that much about sleep apnea. Still, I trusted Kristin would know where to find the cutting-edge treatment. I went back and read all the literature I had on fibromyalgia and sleep. When I read that nearly all fibromyalgia patients suffer from some sleep disorder, I was ready to make the appointment.[5]

Kevin was more easily persuaded than I was.

"You've never slept well in the ten years I've known you," he said. "When I first started working for you, you often complained that you had been up all night because you couldn't sleep."

True. And I had periods where I slept for days at a time. But what if I didn't have a sleep disorder and I was just wasting Lowell's money? Well, that was all I had to lose, someone else's money. I called Stanford and tried to make an appointment, but they wanted a referral from my family doctor.

When I asked my GP for a referral to Stanford, he looked mildly amused. Who was I to demand a referral to the best sleep disorder clinic in the nation? I had a typical case of fibromyalgia. Clinically, I was nobody special. And he didn't take me seriously. Why would Stanford?

"I know your insurance won't pay for this," he said.

"That's okay," I told him. "We're going to pay if the insurance doesn't."

He shrugged and said indifferently, "All right."

Fine by him. I think he was getting tired of me, and he didn't mind referring hypochondriacs from one place to another. If I asked for a referral to a Senegalese witch doctor, he would have sent me, at least just to get rid of me for a while.

A few days later, a receptionist from Stanford called me to make an appointment for a consultation. She said it would take an hour or two and would cost between $400 and $600. If the doctors felt I needed an overnight sleep study, it would cost approximately $5,000.

Well, there went a chunk of Lowell's money. And what would happen if I had the sleep study done and they found nothing?

Two months later, Kevin and I had just sat down in the waiting room on the second floor of the Psychiatry Building at Stanford Medical Clinic when the doctor called my name.

They do that at Stanford. The doctor comes into the waiting room to meet you. You don't have to wait long. The reception room isn't crowded.

---

5   In fact, sleep disorders are a common symptom of FMS.

This doctor looked at me with genuine interest. Because this was a teaching and research hospital, I was not just a patient. I was a specimen. He hoped he would learn something from my illness. I was there because I hoped to benefit from what he had learned from others.

I stood up, clutching my black shoulder bag, which contained my wallet and an old prescription bottle filled with the drugs I always carried with me, including Motrin, aspirin, two Valium, a handful of Vicodin, a couple of antidepressants, and an extra sleeping pill in case of some kind of emergency.

As I followed him down the hall, past the sign that said "Sleep Disorders Clinic," I was certain I was in the wrong place. I didn't have a sleep disorder. I had suffered from fibromyalgia for six years. No one sleeps well when it feels like hot oil is dripping down the spine. At least that's what the fibromyalgia handbooks tell you.

But I was here because I'd been everywhere else. I had lain on my stomach with fine acupuncture needles protruding from my body for hours on end. I had swallowed nutritional supplements at $3 a pill. I had stayed up all night, Googling words like myofascial and guifenesin. I had consulted rheumatologists, neurologists, and herbal specialists.

I had read all the fibromyalgia books. I had faithfully followed their seven-step, twelve-step, or fifteen-step programs. I had taken the drugs my doctors prescribed, religiously filling the little scraps of paper the doctors flung at me as they quickly exited the room. I was here because I had swum, danced, studied Tai Chi, and meditated. Now I was at the end of the road. I had been told dozens of times that my fibromyalgia could be treated, controlled, and even reversed. I had read volumes of magazines, books, Internet articles, and so forth. Their messages were much the same. You can take charge of your pain! You can win this battle! You may even cure this disease if you believe.

If you only believe. That's the telling phrase, the one that tips you off that what's coming is no more effective than the snake oil that nineteenth-century vendors sold. Because you don't have to believe that doctors have removed your appendix for your appendicitis to clear up. You don't have to believe an antibiotic will work for your infection to be cured. You don't have to have faith when you have a wisdom tooth removed. I was here at Stanford not because I still believed, but because, after six years, I couldn't stop trying.

The clock in the examining room read 11:03 when I sat down in the chair next to the wall, the one that the patient always sits in. The doctor didn't sit down. He pulled out the brown manila envelope that held the inch-thick questionnaire I had already completed. He started firing questions at me.

"Ah," he noted.

My sister had a SIDS baby. Any other sudden deaths in my family? What time did I wake up in the morning? Had I ever fallen asleep at the wheel of a car? Did I take afternoon naps? How many hours did I sleep in a day? At 11:09, my back and legs began to cramp up, but he had just begun.

Yes, I did get inexplicably sleepy. Yes, I did have insomnia. But I read the book on fibromyalgia, in fact, dozens of books. Fibromyalgia patients have sleep disorders, including insomnia, wakefulness, and unrefreshing sleep. It was a symptom, not a cause.

It was now 11:30. I was in serious pain, but he wasn't finished. Could he take a picture of my jaw? He pulled out a camera and aimed it at my chin. Could he look in my nose? My throat?

I obediently opened my mouth.

"Kind of crowded in there, isn't it?" he asked.

"Yes."

But I didn't know what he meant. It was the way my mouth had always been. I thought he was commenting on my crooked bottom teeth. Then he asked if another doctor could come in to examine me.

He left the room for a moment and came back with his tall, dark, impeccably groomed colleague. He also looked up my nose and cupped my chin in his hand, turning my head from side to side. Then he sat down across from me.

"I think we can help you," he said.

From his examination, he could see that my jaw and nasal passages were unusually small. As women get older, the muscles inside these passages begin to lose their tautness, and they develop sleep apnea. And lack of sleep from sleep apnea causes muscle contractions, cognitive problems, mood swings, and even bowel and bladder disorders.

I had come to the Sleep Disorders Clinic hoping they would find something wrong, something other than fibromyalgia. In short, I wanted them to find something that could be fixed. But I was amazed that this doctor obviously noticed something extraordinary in five minutes that other doctors hadn't seen in ten years.

"How would this help my fibromyalgia?"

"No matter what you have, if we fix your sleep, you will get better."

I was still suspicious. "What if my medication is causing my sleep problems?"

"We will know that. We will be able to tell how your medications affect your sleep and whether your problems are due to physical obstructions."

Did my sleep apnea have anything to do with my weight? I had only weighed ninety-five pounds in high school. Now I weighed one hundred and thirty-five. Once I was underweight, now I was slightly overweight, and I had added fifteen pounds in the last few years.

"You could lose as much weight as you could, and it wouldn't change anything."

My problem was congenital, a small jaw and narrow nasal passages. As they pointed out with disapproval, I still had my tonsils. I had always been this way, but, as I aged, especially with menopause, the firm muscles in my nose and throat had begun to sag. When I went to sleep, they relaxed completely, restricting or cutting off my air supply.

I was stunned. In my ten-year search for underlying physical conditions that could cause or exacerbate fibromyalgia, I had never thought much about my sleep problems, probably because most fibromyalgia patients have them. As we drove home, I remembered how, as a child, I used to wake up in the night and go to my mother, crying that I couldn't sleep. She thought I had bad dreams, but I knew I didn't. I remembered nights when I had lain awake long after everyone was sleeping, afraid of the car lights reflected on the bedroom walls and the creaking house, while my younger sister slept peacefully beside me.

A few weeks after my visit to Stanford, a sleep study confirmed I had a more than moderate case of sleep apnea. And I did get better. I was fitted with a machine called a controlled positive air pressure (CPAP) with a mask that covers my nose and mouth and blows air down into my lungs. But probably the best news was that I didn't have to go on a raw food diet to get better. I didn't have to give up chocolate or coffee or have my colon cleansed. I didn't even have to believe what they were saying.

Many fibromyalgia patients have underlying conditions that may cause or contribute to their condition. The problem is, as Dr. Rhoades points out, once you are diagnosed with fibromyalgia, some doctors quit looking for answers. You are just one more patient with some confusing, even bizarre, syndrome that can't be fixed or even alleviated. But they are wrong. A diagnosis of a secondary illness or syndrome may not mean that your fibromyalgia can be cured, but, as in my case, it may improve your life more than you had ever dreamed possible.

Of course, not every HMO is going to pay for extensive tests, especially if it doesn't find them relevant. When you are turned down, if you can afford it, you may want to pay for some of these yourself. Unfortunately, we do not, in this country, have anything near approaching equal rights for medical care. But interestingly enough, after the discovery I had sleep apnea, my insurance provider has never balked at paying for my expenses at Stanford.

It cost Lowell nothing, and it has decreased my pain, increased my mental clarity, and, best of all, cured my middle-of-the-night insomnia.

[I]t's long been known that when you stay up all night and are sleep deprived, the amounts of growth hormone and prolactin in your body go down.

Mari Skelly and Andrea Helm,
*Alternative Treatments for Fibromyalgia
& Chronic Fatigue Syndrome*

Chapter Eighteen

Sleep: The Best Therapy

Before my sleep study, I had not slept more than five or six hours a night for a decade. I spent every night from roughly 1:00 to 5:00 AM, wide-awake and reading a book unless I was sedated. The night of my sleep study, I was given my normal ten milligrams of Ambien. In the morning, the technician asked me how many times I had woken up. I looked at him like he was nuts.

"I called you both times I woke up," I said.

He repeated the same question.

"I woke up twice," I said.

When the sleep study results came in the mail, I found I had not awoken twice, as I told the technician, but forty-seven times. Not only that, I had only been asleep for two hundred and eighty-eight minutes all night, a total of 4.8 hours. The rest of the time, another one hundred and forty minutes, I was unconscious, but my sleep was so extremely light that, technically, I was awake. During the time I was clinically asleep, I had woken up over ten times an hour.

Even more astounding, or perhaps predictable, was the fact that nearly all my arousals came between 12:30 and 4:00 AM, the same exact time that my nightly nocturnal awakenings began and ended. I woke up restless, anxious, and depressed in the middle of the night, not because I was stressed, but because I was having trouble breathing.

The Stanford doctors were also right. I had no central nervous system apneas, which meant my sleep problems had nothing to do with a faulty nervous system or medication. Every time I woke up, it corresponded to a breathing obstruction.

Kevin was jubilant. At last, the doctors had found something that could be treated. I was astonished and, at the same time, not surprised. I was astonished because I had, on one hand, been so convinced that I did not have a sleep disorder. Yet, when I looked back at my sleeping patterns throughout my life, it should have been easy for me to see. Why did I miss it? I was born with it, and the symptoms came on so gradually over the course of my life. But how had all the doctors missed it?

The best news was the insurance paid for my treatment. Because I was in an HMO, my family doctor had to get an approval for further treatment of my sleep apnea. I thought my family doctor might be interested in the results of my sleep study, if nothing else than to hear about Stanford's recent progress in establishing a link between sleep disorders and fibromyalgia, but, when I went to him, he didn't have much to say. I asked him how, after seeing twenty doctors or more, all of them could have missed the diagnosis of sleep apnea, especially when my initial complaints, long before I developed fibromyalgia, were insomnia and excessive daytime sleepiness.

"You don't fit the pattern," he said. "You're not male. You're not obese."

He shrugged as if to say, "How would I know?"

"I thought doctors were supposed to diagnose," I said to Kevin later. "It seems that, if you don't fit some kind of stereotype, they can't find out what's wrong with you. Even I could figure out an overweight male might have sleep apnea or a menopausal woman might be stressed."

◆   ◆   ◆

Once again, Stanford's clinic couldn't fit me in for months, but, a few weeks later, the receptionist called to tell me they had a cancellation at 2:00 PM that day. It was a three-hour drive. Before I could awaken Kevin to tell him the news, the phone rang again. The receptionist was also scheduling me for a second sleep study that night, in case the doctor prescribed a breathing machine for me. If that happened, the technicians would have to hook me up to the device and monitor my sleep for a full night to determine the correct pressure. They would do the sleep study that same night.

"So you're telling me to bring an overnight bag?" I asked.

"Yes," she said. "Just in case."

I figured "just in case" was a pretty sure thing. I knew I was getting a CPAP, but I had a million questions that I fired at the doctors.

How did they know that my pain wasn't causing my sleeping problems? They showed me how my awakenings corresponded to a drop in oxygen in every case. Neither the pain nor any of the drugs I was taking were affecting my sleep.

"Your brain works very well," the specialist said. "Whenever your oxygen rate dips below 90 percent, your brain has to make a decision. What does it want to do? Continue to sleep or wake up so you can take a deep breath? In every case, your brain chose breathing over sleeping."

"How would improving my sleep affect my fibromyalgia?"

"No matter what's wrong with you right now, you will get better. Improving your sleep will help your brain improve the way it processes pain."

"So would you say I had a minor case of sleep apnea?"

He frowned. "No, I wouldn't say that at all."

"A moderate case?"

"It's definitely well into moderate. Not the worst case we have seen, but it's certainly well beyond moderate."

I had other questions, too many, but I was looking forward to the night when they would monitor me as I slept with a mask for the first time with the same enthusiasm that young women used to look forward to their wedding nights.

What would it be like to sleep, dream, and perhaps wake in the morning feeling like I hadn't been walked on all night by a pair of flat-footed gnomes? I couldn't wait to get the CPAP mask on. I never wanted to sleep without it again.

I had been worried about sleeping with a mask because I am claustrophobic. But, with the promise of even minor improvement, my anxiety changed to excitement. I felt like I was getting a crown. I was elated as the technician fitted me with two sets of straps, one around the forehead and another around the chin, holding a large, obtrusive plastic muzzle in place. At the top, in the area of the eyebrows, a large vent allowed the exhaled air to escape. Basically, it looks like a gas mask, and it is attached to a machine with a long, gray tube three inches in circumference.

Sure, I didn't look good in my mask, but the thought of sudden death put an immediate end to my vanity. And even if it wasn't comfortable, after six years of chronic pain, how distressing could it be?

An hour later, I was lying flat on my back while she turned the machine on. "At first it will feel like you can't exhale. But just go ahead and do it anyway."

Then the wind blew into my lungs. Your chest blows up with air. And I did feel like I wouldn't be able to get the air back out. But it was surprisingly easy to breathe against it. As the technician predicted, I struggled with the mask all night. I pulled it off three or four times, and she came in to wake me up and tell me to put it back on.

Finally at 5:00 AM, she came in to tell me I could take it off. "Just rest now."

I dozed for about a half hour and then woke up again. I rang and asked her to put the mask back on. Her dire words about sudden death had made me very attached to my little machine. I didn't want to sleep without it, even for an hour.

When I first woke up, I felt a bit better. I still had the head-to-toe pain, but I felt a little rested. I put it down to a placebo effect. I had expected to feel better, and I did.

I had a follow-up appointment six weeks after I started using my CPAP. I should feel a big improvement in my daily activities over the next three months, and, if I did, I was to be sure to call and let him know.

"We like to know that," he said.

A few days later, for the first time in years, I woke up without pain. I lay there for a minute without comprehending what was happening.

"Something's different," I thought.

I stretched my legs. Yep, they were still there. They just didn't burn like fire. I moved my arms and my shoulders. Everything worked. It was like someone had come in during the night and oiled all my joints. Only when I moved my neck from side to side did I feel twinges of pain.

I also felt a little drowsy. Drowsy was also something I hadn't experienced in years. I generally went from sleeping to wide-awake, from

Why GP's Don't Get It

"The sheer volume of information that underpins modern medicine … continues to increase at an exponential rate. The physician is between a rock and a hard place, with society crying out for a level of care that most physicians want desperately to provide but often find they cannot. Nowhere is this more evident than in the treatment of modern pain."

Arthur Rosenfeld,
The Truth about Chronic Pain

unconscious to consciousness of pain. Drowsy was a welcome world in between.

When I looked in the mirror, my face was pink. I had never noticed how pale it was before.

For about an hour, I thought perhaps I was cured, but, as I got dressed and started sweeping and unloading the dishwasher, the old, familiar pain returned, except it was much weaker. It was maybe a five on a scale of one to ten. I took my pain pills, and they worked. By now, I was down to a two on the scale.

By night, however, I was really hurting again. Over the next six weeks, I rode the pain escalator up and down. I never got to the first floor, but I never got higher than nine, even though the escalator went up to the tenth floor.

You would have thought I was elated, and some days I was. But pain is relative. The better I felt, the better I wanted to feel. The more good days I had, the more I realized that most of my days for the last ten years had been very bad. I felt like I had lost a large chunk of my life. I was impatient.

I was also anxious. Most of the time, I had tried something new—from magnets to massage—the therapy seemed to work at first, and then, once again, pain would overtake me. I felt like my disease was an enemy plotting against me, huddling up in my spine while I tossed and turned, figuring out a way to overcome the benefits of magnets and massage, and leaving me debilitated once again.

So I waited, thinking that, any day, the pain would return like a giant wave crashing as the tide comes in, flooding the damp shore. When I had a bad day, which now meant a base pain of seven or, on a rare occasion, an eight, I was sure the pain was building up again.

Sleeping with a CPAP was interesting. The doctor told me that, after a while, my body would adjust to it and even prefer it because, subconsciously, I would recognize its benefits.

Painless awakenings didn't happen often those first six weeks. They came about once every ten days. But I sometimes wake up in pain, only to find that it diminished in the afternoon.

By now, I was sure there was something more I needed to control the pain, something besides pain pills, massages, stress-free days, exercise, or meditation. And that something was sleep.

I was having nice dreams, not ethereal, heavenly dreams, but vivid dreams generally related to what was going on in my life. They were childlike dreams.

Six weeks later, I was back at Stanford for my first checkup. Yes, I was getting better, but it was slow. Very slow. And bad days, which were once much more common and severe, became intolerable. Pain is, after all, relative. Two or three doctors were in the room with me for over an hour, asking questions I couldn't answer, like "Would you say you're sleepier or more fatigued?" I was both. Who knew which came first?

They were elated to hear I had improved already, even if I was impatient and dissatisfied. But I wanted an answer to the big question. Had anyone ever recovered completely from fibromyalgia after he or she was treated for sleep apnea?

"Will I be able to go back to work?" I asked.

The head doctor answered this one. The stress of a job would interfere with the progress I was making. I shouldn't go back to work until I was sleeping well most of the time. That would be a while, if ever.

"Weeks? Months? Years?"

Well, they really hadn't been studying this for years, and nobody really recovered in weeks. Months, lots of months. Maybe years. Maybe never.

"Come back in three months," they told me.

"Well," I told myself, "you can't have everything."

It was getting easier to settle for what I could have, a reduction in pain, more pleasant nights, and more energy. I sometimes woke up feeling nearly free of pain. That delicious feeling only lasted ten minutes or so, but it was a blissful ten minutes. For years, I had dreamed of five minutes without pain. It was just five minutes, enough to clear my mind. Now I knew how it felt, like a loud, unpleasant background noise had been switched off. It was as if a booming stereo blasting the type of music you hate the most right into your eardrum had been unplugged. It was quiet. It was sensual. It was nice. But sleeping with a CPAP didn't fix as much as I hoped.

It's been two years since I started my sleep therapy. I'd love to say I'm completely well. I'm not. It's unlikely I will ever be. No test can tell if I have permanent neurological damage from all those years without sleep or some other problem. Somewhere, a pain switch may have been triggered that can't be turned off, making me overly sensitive to mild discomfort, like riding in a car for hours at a time.

During good times, I ride my bicycle and exercise. I wake up some mornings feeling rested. Most days, my husband can put his hand on my knee, and I don't have to ask him to move it. Noise irritates me less. At one time, I hated to go to the movies because the volume seemed to be so loud that it physically hurt. Now it doesn't bother me as much.

I am reaching out to other people and making new friends. I chose my friends more carefully. I don't have as much mental disorientation. When it comes on, I can recognize it. I refer to it now as "one of my spells." These spells usually last a few hours and are similar in some ways to a migraine, except I don't have a headache. Everything gets a little blurry around the edges. I try not to drive when I feel one coming on. In fact, I generally get a good book and read or watch television until it passes. I try not to handle things like checkbooks or keys so I don't misplace them. I tell Kevin, which is really important, because I get very frustrated sometimes when he is trying to have a serious discussion about money or a trip and I am having trouble focusing.

On a less positive sign, several months after my sleep treatment began, I started to menstruate again. Now fifty-nine, I can't say I am particularly pleased. But I suppose it is a sign of good health.

Every day I try to weigh what I can do versus what I want to do. I try to do important things first, in case I run out of energy or have to reach for the heavy-duty pain medicine. I have a better sense of what is important in my life.

Because my symptoms fluctuate on a weekly, daily, or hourly basis, I can't expect to go back to work. I use a different standard now to judge my worth. As I lie in bed at night, I ask myself what I have done to make someone's life easier that day.

But when the doctors discovered I had sleep apnea, I began to realize that there may be some FMS patients who are misdiagnosed. Only a battery of tests and a round of consultations can confirm that. If I could do it all over again, from the minute I was diagnosed with fibromyalgia, I would have insisted on tests to rule out every possible disorder that could have affected, irritated, or caused fibromyalgia. In addition to a sleep study, I would have asked for a brain scan and cardiopulmonary tests. I would have had an MRI of my spinal column. I would do all these things to make sure some GP hadn't taken a look at me and decided I fit the profile for fibromyalgia.

Once you have been diagnosed with fibromyalgia, you may find that every symptom you have, including side effects from medicine or other medical problems, will be attributed to FMS. Recently, my sister, who has had fibromyalgia for two decades, has been diagnosed with Parkinson's disease as well. She is already troubled with some symptoms that typically don't appear until a few years after the disease is discovered.

"I think I've had Parkinson's for about six years," she said.

That's when she started having tremors and began to walk with an odd gait. Doctors said she might have had a stroke, but the tremors and other symptoms were never fully investigated. Parkinson's disease is a serious disorder that needs to be treated aggressively, the sooner the better. Patients with fibromyalgia are seriously at risk because doctors often lump together all sorts of symptoms that may be indicative of other problems.[6]

Every time I read a well-intended book on treating fibromyalgia, I wince as the author passes over sleep disorders without recommending a sleep study. Even if sleep apnea is not the underlying cause of fibromyalgia, it is possible to have fibromyalgia that may be connected with trouble breathing that keeps you from sound sleep.

If you have fibromyalgia, keep going and keep searching. Get a different opinion and a different perspective. Somewhere out there, there is an answer or answers. There are medications to relieve some pain, exercises to keep your muscles from tightening, and meditations to help your peace of mind.

Sometimes, when I'm dancing, watching a sunset, or playing with my grandchildren, I am glad I survived the days and nights of intense pain and despair created by mental confusion. It was all worth it to have one good day.

Dr. Rhoades believes patients who exhibit fibromyalgia symptoms usually have some sort of trauma. He explains:

Clearly something has gone wrong with the transmission in the nervous system, whether it is a result of trauma or sleep apnea or a myr-

---

6   Of course, because some of her medications can cause Parkinson's symptoms, we can't be sure that she really has Parkinson's. This is why an experienced doctor who specializes in fibromyalgia is essential.

iad of other conditions. We can try a number of approaches. Hopefully we find an underlying condition we can treat. And we have to try to soothe the nervous system, which has become so over-excited it changes innocuous signals into pain. I think this pain stems from an irregularity in the limbic system, but, as I said, all we can do right now is to improve the quality of life.

Often patients reject drugs because they have been told they will become addicted. Many patients come to me because their physicians have refused to give them more pain medicine. Many are confused about what pain drugs will do for them.

And patients may need to be treated with more than just drugs. In many cases, physical therapy is appropriate; injections may be helpful for certain problems. But when a patient tells me he or she is in pain, I have no reason not to believe them unless proven otherwise.

Physicians have to be careful about stereotyping patients; sometimes it's hard not to do. Age, social position, education—these all play a role in who the patient is. But if you believe your patient, they will believe in you, and that's an important part of motivating your patient to comply with treatment.

Doctors and patients should not be at odds: We both want the same thing: better health for the patient and better quality of life.

Trust your doctor to decide which set of tests is best in your case to ensure no other medical problems are present. This will help you avoid extra testing that will add little to your diagnosis and only add expense.

Harris H. McIlwain, MD,
and Debra Fulghum Bruce,
*Fibromyalgia Handbook:
A 7-Step Program to Halt
and Even Reverse Fibromyalgia*

Chapter Nineteen

Getting a Complete Diagnosis

Fibromyalgia is a junk diagnosis. If you have been diagnosed with it, you may not have it. You may have it, but still haven't been diagnosed. You may have an underlying condition, as I did, that is causing or contributing to your fibromyalgia. Fibromyalgia specialist Dr. Brown wrote in *Alternative Treatments for Fibromyalgia & Chronic Pain Syndrome* that eleven of forty-six women diagnosed with fibromyalgia didn't have it.

If you have been diagnosed with fibromyalgia, chances are you have been dumped into the soup of patients with incurable disorders. Because it isn't an incurable disorder with a life-or-death outcome, like cancer, the GP will prescribe pills that were recommended by a colleague, another patient, or, worse yet, his drug rep.

No more tests. No more referrals. You'll come back on a regular basis, and the doctor will listen just long enough to justify his fee. If you're no worse, the doctor will refill the same prescriptions. If you're worse, the doctor will increase the dosage or switch to another medicine. Or maybe not. Maybe he or she will just ask if you're exercising. Maybe he or she will tell you to take off some weight. Or maybe you'll just get the lecture about positive thinking, learning to live with it, and quitting complaining.

When I asked the technician who strapped on the monitor for my sleep study what would have happened if I hadn't come all the way to Stanford and doctors had never found my sleep apnea, she said dispassionately, almost cheerfully, "You would have died."

And it's true. People of all ages die all the time of undiagnosed sleep apnea. Most of the time, they have heart attacks or strokes in their sleep, so you won't see sleep apnea listed as the cause of death. If the deceased is, as I am, a woman of average weight, her death will be linked to heart disease or maybe high blood pressure.

What happened to the woman who died alone in her mobile home, the one who underlined all those pep talks, the one who spent her last dollars on expensive vitamin supplements and glossy books on curing or containing the disease? Did she overdose? Or did she have a heart attack? I hate to think it was sleep apnea, something that could have been treated with a CPAP. This might have reversed her symptoms. If you have fibromyalgia, don't let this happen to you.

Fibromyalgia patients are often neglected, misunderstood, misdiagnosed, and mistreated. It is estimated that 3 to 5 percent of the population have fibromyalgia, yet there is still no specialist to treat it. Whether you are diagnosed with it or think you might have it, you have to take your treatment into your own hands. Remember the following:

Doctors Can Be Inconsistent

What one doctor may diagnose as chronic bursitis, arthritis, or even a slipped disk, another will call fibromyalgia. I have three sisters. Two have been diagnosed with fibromyalgia. One has classic symptoms, including pain in all four quadrants of the body, sleep problems, memory problems, and problems with bladder control. My younger sister, on the other hand, has chronic neck pain. When she told us she had scar tissue from fibromyalgia, we wondered, "How could that be?" I had never found scar tissue mentioned in any of the texts I had read. She has had surgery on her neck. When she confronted her doctor, he told her that doctors diagnose fibromyalgia differently. What is fibromyalgia to one physician is something else to another.

The National Arthritis Association (NAA) has attempted to identify the symptoms, including widespread pain affecting the left and right side of the body, above and below the waist, that have persisted for at least three months, with pain on digital palpation in at least eleven of eighteen specified tender points when four kilograms of force (or nine pounds of pressure, enough to whiten the fingernail) is applied. The points cluster around the neck, shoulder, chest, hip, knee, elbow, and in places where the muscle narrows and attaches to the bone. Did my sister meet those criteria? No, she did not.

And notice that the definition of FMS by the NAA does not include morning stiffness, fatigue, sleep disturbance, confusion, or any of the other symptoms generally ascribed to FMS.

In his book, *Complications*, surgeon Atul Gawande discusses at length the lack of consistency between medical opinions, even when the disease, such as gall bladder disease, is common and well-defined. One of Dr. Gawande's resources is Jack Wennberg and his research team, who have studied decision-making in medicine across the country.[7] Gawande writes:

> What he (Wennberg) has found is a stubborn, over-whelming, and embarrassing degree of inconsistency in what we do. His research has shown, for example, that the likelihood of a doctor sending you for a gall-bladder-removal operation varies 270 percent depending on what city you live in; for a hip replacement, 450 percent; for care in an intensive care unit during the last six months of your life, 880 percent. A patient in Santa Barbara, California, is five time more likely to be recommended for back surgery for a back pain than one in Bronx, New York. This is, in the main, uncertainty at work, with the varying experiences, habits, and intuitions of individual doctors leading to massively different care for different people.

Scary, isn't it? I used to think getting a second opinion was playing it safe. Now I think it's just as likely that two doctors can be wrong. If doctors can't agree over a relatively well-understood condition such as gall bladder disease and when it necessitates an operation, how many will correctly diagnose fibromyalgia?

You have to become an expert at how the disease is assessed so you can gauge the likelihood that you have the disorder. And get a second and third opinion. Talk to other fibromyalgia patients.

Sometimes, in an effort to deal with these inconsistencies, doctors talk about subsets of fibromyalgia, especially when they are trying to identify causes or triggers. Find out what subset you belong to. Did

---

7   Wennberg's findings are available online at www.dartmouthatlas.org.

yours come on after trauma, such as a car accident? Did an illness trigger it?

However, keep in mind that, just because you had a car accident a year or two before you developed symptoms, it doesn't necessarily mean the accident caused your fibromyalgia. Popular theories about causes and treatments for fibromyalgia come and go. In the last few weeks, a couple of well-meaning friends have told me that taking vitamin D will cure or help contain the symptoms of fibromyalgia. Where this idea originated, I don't know.

But if you have fibromyalgia or suspect you do, don't take your doctor's word for it. Find out what your doctor means, and, more importantly, what he means to do about it.

Doctors Are Often Wrong

It's almost sacrilege to say doctors are wrong in the United States, where most people dislike doctors as a group but trust their own implicitly. In *Complications*, Dr. Gawande writes:

> How often do autopsies turn up a major misdiagnosis in the cause of death? I would have guessed this happened rarely, in 1 or 2 percent of cases at most. According to three studies done in 1998 and 1999, however, the figure is about 40 percent. A large review of autopsy studies concluded that in about a third of the misdiagnoses the patients would have been expected to live if proper treatment had been administered. George Lundberg, a pathologist and former editor of the *Journal of American Medicine*, has done more than anyone to call attention to these figures. He points out the most surprising fact of all: the rates at which misdiagnosis is detected in autopsy studies have not improved since 1938.

With all the recent advances in imaging and diagnostics, it's hard to accept that we not only get the diagnosis wrong in two out of five of our patients who die but we have also failed to improve over time. To see if this really could be true, doctors at Harvard put together a simple study.

They went back to their hospital records to see how often autopsies picked up missed diagnoses in 1960 and 1970, before the advent of the CT, ultrasound, nuclear scanning, and other technologies, and then in 1980, after those technologies became widely used. The researchers found no improvement. Regardless of the decade, the physicians missed a quarter of fatal infections, a third of heart attacks, and almost two-thirds of pulmonary emboli in their patients who died.

In most cases, technology didn't fail. Rather, the physicians did not consider the correct diagnosis in the first place. The perfect test or scan might have been available, but the physician never ordered it.

Granted, as Dr. Gawande points out, a correct diagnosis is not as simple as most laymen would like to believe. The course of disease in the human body can be more perplexing than predicting the path of a hurricane. A GP who sees only a few FMS patients in a week or a month is unlikely to know or understand the subtleties of the syndrome or know FMS has been linked to sleep disorders, neurological damage, muscle tissue abnormalities including hypoxemia (insufficient oxygen) and ischemia (decreased blood flow), anti-immune disorders, viruses and bacterial infections, abnormal levels of hormones, thyroid disorders, brain scan abnormalities, neurotransmitter disorders, chronic fatigue syndrome, post-traumatic stress disorder, abnormal steroid levels, or pain processing by the central nervous system.

Another Twelve-step Tip

Sometimes, no matter what the problem, we have to take one day at a time, one hour at a time and even one minute at a time.

All patients diagnosed with FMS should request blood tests to rule out anemia, thyroid disorder, rheumatoid arthritis, and lupus. They should ask for a brain scan to rule out MS. They should visit a rheumatologist who will be able to distinguish fibromyalgia from other crippling illnesses, like arthritis and gout. They should visit a pain specialist who is willing to help them find some relief from their suffering. They should also get a sleep study. I believe that mine probably saved my life.

This list is not meant to be exhaustive. There is no doubt that other tests that should be done, depending on how your symptoms are affecting you. If your pain stems from your back and shoots down your arms and legs, you may need x-rays or a CAT scan to check for a herniated disc.

As for the self-help books, they are confusing and contradictory and dispense the same, tired clichés, as if a prayer book, a handful of mustard greens and rutabaga, and some good, old-fashioned exercise will kick the disease right out of your body. These books will make you feel better at first, but, when you fail to cure yourself, you will feel worse. You will believe it was your lack of will, that is, your inability to give up steak or mashed potatoes or ice cream. It was your negative thinking. Doesn't your husband tell you that you complain all the time? It was your financial position. Who can afford those vitamins at $200 a month?

But many of them also contain some excellent background information if you haven't seriously studied FMS. *Chronic Fatigue Syndrome, Fibromyalgia and Other Invisible Illnesses,* by Katrina Berne, PhD, provides a thorough discussion of how fibromyalgia is defined and a list of other diseases with which it may be confused. The quarterly magazine, *Fibromyalgia Network,* edited by Kristin Thorson, keeps up with current research and scientific literature and presents it in understandable layman's terms.

There are support groups in person or online. I would certainly advise you to check them out. I've never found a good one, however. Unless a health professional monitors them, these meetings often descend into whining and self-pity too often for my taste. As much as I don't like overly exuberant expectations, I dislike despair and a sense of helplessness even more. I have spent years trying to balance my hope for the future against the realities of my illness. I may be sick, but I also want to be sane.

It's difficult to find physicians who want to treat fibromyalgia. If you can't find a fibromyalgia expert in your area, your best bet is probably a pain specialist. My pain specialist, as I've mentioned before, says that pain doctors generally see the patients no one else wants to see. Their doctors have often given up on them. Dr. Rhoades concentrates on what is going to make them comfortable. If patients tell him they have tried a specific treatment and have not found it to be effective, he will try something else. He doesn't discourage patients from trying alternative treatments, including homeopathy, vitamin supplements, and so forth. He offers pain medication when appropriate, but doesn't try to force any particular treatment on patients. He says he listens to them, often a rarity in the medical profession, and tends to believe what they tell him until proven otherwise.

"Sometimes I am surprised by what patients say other physicians have told them about their condition, but it is not my job to argue over a particular diagnosis. It's my job to improve the quality of life for my patients. Instead of confronting, I listen to my patients and let them tell me what they feel has been effective and what has not. Relieving pain means coming up with the right formula for each patient, and only they can tell me what they are feeling."

It should be noted that certain drug therapies for fibromyalgia may worsen obstructive sleep apnea and actually exacerbate the patient's symptoms of fatigue and restless sleep.

Harris H. McIlwain, MD,
and Debra Fulgham Bruce,
*The Fibromyalgia Handbook:
A 7-Step Program to Halt
and Even Reverse Fibromyalgia*

Chapter Twenty

The Dangers to Your Health You Can't Ignore

Fibromyalgia is not fatal. That's what the experts say. You won't die of crippling pain, fatigue, and mental confusion. You won't see fibromyalgia on an autopsy report. But you may die of related causes. If you have fibromyalgia, you need to guard against the fatal consequences of intractable pain, stress, lack of sleep, and mental confusion, including these:

Accidental Overdose or Side Effect of Drugs

If you are visiting one or two doctors, they may prescribe drugs that aren't compatible. In fact, your own doctor may forget what he or she has already prescribed. I always ask, "Now will this new drug affect the Vicodin and sleep medication that I'm already on?" You would be surprised how many times the doctor has to pick up my chart and

---

If You Need Legal Help

If you want to keep your job and your employer is uncooperative, check out the Patient Advocacy Foundation at (800) 532-5274 or online at www.patientadvocacy.org

---

rifle through the pages, reviewing what he has already prescribed. Certain types of antidepressants can be fatal if taken together. When my doctor prescribed methadone, she did not tell me to quit taking my other pain medications. Of course, it was obvious to me, but might not have been on one of the days when I wasn't thinking clearly.

The son of the late Anna Nicole Smith died of low doses of antidepressants and methadone. Several of the drugs you may be taking, including antidepressants and opioids, cannot be discontinued without a doctor's supervision. Make sure you know what ones these are and always consult your doctor before you discontinue a drug.

Some drugs may be dangerous if you have undiagnosed sleep apnea or heart condition. Be sure to get a stress test and a sleep study done. I know most doctors won't see a need for a stress test or an EKG, but if you are taking heavy doses or even light doses of numerous drugs, you want to be sure your cardiopulmonary functions are at their best.

Get a plastic case and portion out your medication every day. I resisted this for a long time because it seemed like something only senile, old people would do. But many days I had to guess if I had taken my medication or not.

Intractable Pain

Yes, it can kill you. Every time my pain gets about a certain level, my blood pressure soars. It's been as high as 210/120. That's stroke and heart attack territory.

Overwork

This is also an invitation to heart attack, stroke, or even a serious virus. You have a serious condition. Treat it seriously. Don't be pressured by glib advice to get your mind off the pain. Rest is still one of the highest-rated therapies by patients who rate therapies themselves. Don't feel guilty.

Despair

In literature, lovers die of unrequited love all the time. Doctors who don't believe this will shake their heads after a patient dies and say, "I dunno. They just gave up."

This is the time to make yourself as happy as you possibly can. My favorite things are bubble baths, aromatic candles, fresh flowers, sunshine, the beach, silly romantic movies, good books and magazines, John Coltrane CDs, and hearing my grandchildren tell me about school.

Pamper yourself whenever you can. Be absolutely selfish. Ask someone to bring you a cup of tea or make you some chicken soup. Sing off-key along with a karaoke CD, or, if you are well enough, take singing lessons. If you really feel you can't go on, why not indulge any whim or passion you've ever had? In fact, probably the only good thing about the suffering, from my perspective, is that I learned to enjoy myself to whatever extent I was able to do so.

Missed Diagnosis

If you suspect you have fibromyalgia and your doctor doesn't agree, by all means get a second or third opinion. Some doctors still don't believe in FMS. If your doctor dismisses your pain or believes you are a malingerer, get another doctor. On average, patients have fibromyalgia for six years before they are diagnosed. Don't be one of them.

Wrong Diagnosis and Treatment

If you are diagnosed with fibromyalgia, make certain you get the complete battery of tests to rule out other conditions. You need a blood panel, a sleep study, a thyroid test, a brain scan, and a neurological study. Don't be satisfied until you have ruled out anything that may be contributing to or causing your pain.

Mental Confusion

Be careful driving. Take maps with you whenever you go somewhere new. Be careful with your medication. You may want to have someone else monitor it for you. If you are taking a new drug, have someone check up on you.

Suicide

If these other conditions don't get to you first, you may decide it's not worth it anyway. Remember, scientists may find a new treatment for fibromyalgia next week. You don't want to be the last one who killed themselves waiting.

Discuss your feelings with your doctors and your family. If necessary, take drastic measures, like a change in medication, go on a trip, or do something extravagant. I once spent a whole day shopping for clothes because I decided that, if I was going to die, I might as well spend some money first. I might add that I've worn the clothes often and I've never been sorry. Why worry about a little credit card debt if you feel like you're dying anyway?

Remember what my pain doctor said. "I'm sure we are on the verge of finding a way to treat fibromyalgia. The trick is keeping patients alive long enough for it to benefit them."

I've written this book because I felt fibromyalgia isn't being taken seriously enough. I think a fibromyalgia patient deserves something more than a platitude like "eat your vegetables." And I do think there are better answers out there, even today.

I wanted to tell everyone about the words that changed my life. "I want you to find the best treatment for fibromyalgia." Find the best doctors you can, physicians you are compatible with. Learn all you can about your condition. Make life as livable as you can.

Recommended Reading

Bennett, R.M. et al. 1989. Beyond fibromyalgia: ideas on etiology and treatment. *Journal of Rheumatology* 16:185.

Beinfield, Harriett, LAc, and Efrem Korngold, LAc, OMD. *Between Heaven and Earth: A Guide to Chinese Medicine.* New York: Ballantine Books, 1992.

Blakeslee, Sandra, and Matthew Blakeslee. *The Body Has a Mind of Its Own.* New York: Random House, 2007.

Cunningham, Chet. *The Fibromyalgia Relief Handbook.* Encintas: United Research Publishers, 2003.

National Institute of Arthritis & Musculoskelatal and Skin Diseases Web site: http://www.niams.nih.gov

Gawande, Atul. *Complications.* New York: Metropolitan Books: Henry Holt, 2002.

Gyatso, Geshe Kelsang. *Meditation Handbook.* Ulverston, England: Tharpa Publications, 1995.

Haas, Elson M., MD. *Staying Healthy with the Seasons.* Berkeley: Celestial Arts, 1981.

Horstman, Judith. *The Arthritis Foundation's Guide to Alternative Therapies.* Atlanta: The Arthritis Foundation, 1999.

Kaptchuk, Ted J. *The Web That Has No Weaver: Understanding Chinese Medicine.* New York: Congdon & Weed, 1993.

Nurland, Sherwin, *The Wisdom of the Body.* New York: Knopf, 1997.

Pellegrino, Mark, MD. *Fibromyalgia: Managing the Pain.* Columbus: Anadem Publishing, 1993.

———. *The Fibromyalgia Survivor.* Columbus: Anadem Publishing, 1995.

———. *Inside Fibromyalgia.* Columbus: Anadem Publishing, 2001.

Rosenfeld, Arthur. *The Truth about Chronic Pain.* New York: Basic Books, 2003.

Rybacki, James J., PharmD, and James W. Long, MD. *The Essential Guide to Prescription Drugs*. New York, HarperPerennial, 1996.

Skelly, Mari, and Andrea Helm. *Alternative Treatment for Fibromyalgia & Chronic Fatigue Syndrome*. Alameda: Hunter House, 1999.

Starlanyl, Devin, and Mary Ellen Copeland. *Fibromyalgia and Chronic Myofascial Pain Syndrome: A Survival Manual*. Oakland: New Harbinger, 1996.

Starlanyl, Devin. *The Fibromyalgia Advocate*. Oakland: New Harbinger, 1999.

Teitelbaum, Jacob, MD. *Pain Free 1-2-3*. New York: McGraw-Hill, 2005.

Williamson, Miriam Ehrlich, and David A. Nye. *Fibromyalgia: A Comprehensive Approach*. New York: Walker Publishing, 1996.

Other References

Berne, Katrina. *Chronic Fatigue Syndrome, Fibromyalgia and other Invisible Symptoms*. Alameda: Hunter House, 2002.
———. *Running on Empty: The Complete Guide to Chronic Fatigue Syndrome*. Hunter House, 1995.
Elrod, Joe M. *Reversing Fibromyalgia*. New York: Walker Publishing, 1996.
Fransen, Jenny, and I. Jon Russell. *The Fibromyalgia Help Book: A Practical Guide to Living Better with Fibromyalgia*. St. Paul: Smith House Press, 1996.
McIlwain, Harris H., MD, and Debra Fulghum Bruce. *The Fibromyalgia Handbook: A 7-Step Treatment to Halt and Even Reverse Fibromyalgia*. New York: Henry Holt & Company, 1996.
Kelly, Julie, Rosalie Devonshire, and Thomas Romaro. *Taking Charge of Fibromyalgia*. Wayzata: Fibromyalgia Education Systems Inc., 2005.
Kidson, Ruth. *Acupuncture for Everyone*. Rochester: Healing Arts Press, 2000.
Lidell, Lucinda, with Sara Thomas, Carola Beresford Cooke, and Anthony Porter. *The Book of Massage*. New York: Gaia Books, 1984.
Matallana, Lynne, Laurence Bradley, Stuart Silverman, and Muhammad Yumus. *A Complete Idiot's Guide to Fibromyalgia*. New York: Alpha Books, 2005.
McIlwain, Harris H., MD, and Debra Fulghum Bruce. *The Fibromyalgia Handbook: A 7-Step Program to Halt and Even Reverse Fibromyalgia*. New York: Henry Holt, 1999.
Merek, Claudia Craig. *The First Year: Fibromyalgia: An Essential Guide for the Newly Diagnosed*. New York: Marlowe & Company, 2003.

Reed, Daniel, *The Complete Book of Chinese Health and Healing: Guarding the Three Treasures*. Boston: Shambhala, 1995.

Rubin Jordan. *The Great Physician's RX: 7 Weeks of Wellness Success Guide*. Nashville: Thomas Nelson Publishing, 2006.

St. Armand, R. Paul, MD, and Claudia Craig Marek. *What Your Doctor May Not Tell You About Fibromyalgia*. New York: Warner Books, 2003.

Teitelbaum, Jacob, MD. *From Fatigued to Fantastic!* New York: Avery, 2001.

———. *Pain Free 1-2-3*. New York: McGraw-Hill, 2005.

WITHDRAWN

CPSIA information can be obtained at www.ICGtesting.com
Printed in the USA
LVOW061723030112

262215LV00003B/114/P